Counseling
and Psychotherapy
with College Students

Counseling and Psychotherapy with College Students

A Guide to Treatment

Edited by
Joseph E. Talley
and
W.J. Kenneth Rockwell

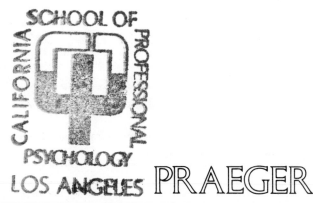

PRAEGER SPECIAL STUDIES • PRAEGER SCIENTIFIC

New York • Philadelphia • Eastbourne, UK
Toronto • Hong Kong • Tokyo • Sydney

Library of Congress Cataloging-in-Publication Data
Main entry under title:

Counseling and psychotherapy with college students.

Includes bibliographies and index.
1. College students — Mental health services.
2. College students — Counseling of. 3. Psychotherapy.
I. Talley, Joseph E. II. Rockwell, W. J. Kenneth.
[DNLM: 1. Counseling. 2. Psychotherapy. 3. Student
Health Services. WA 353 C855]
RC451.4.S7C684 1985   378'.1946   85-16957
ISBN 0-03-004654-8 (alk. paper)

Published in 1986 by Praeger Publishers
CBS Educational and Professional Publishing, a Division of CBS Inc.
521 Fifth Avenue, New York, NY 10175 USA

© 1986 by Praeger Publishers

6789   052   987654321

Printed in the United States of America on acid-free paper

INTERNATIONAL OFFICES

Orders from outside the United States should be sent to the appropriate address listed below. Orders from areas not listed below should be placed through CBS International Publishing, 383 Madison Ave., New York, NY 10175 USA

Australia, New Zealand
Holt Saunders, Pty. Ltd., 9 Waltham St., Artarmon, N.S.W. 2064, Sydney, Australia

Canada
Holt, Rinehart & Winston of Canada, 55 Horner Ave., Toronto, Ontario, Canada M8Z 4X6

Europe, the Middle East, & Africa
Holt Saunders, Ltd., 1 St. Anne's Road, Eastbourne, East Sussex, England BN21 3UN

Japan
Holt Saunders, Ltd., Ichibancho Central Building, 22-1 Ichibancho, 3rd Floor, Chiyodaku, Tokyo, Japan

Hong Kong, Southeast Asia
Holt Saunders Asia, Ltd., 10 Fl. Intercontinental Plaza, 94 Granville Road, Tsim Sha Tsui East, Kowloon, Hong Kong

Manuscript submissions should be sent to the Editorial Director, Praeger Publishers, 521 Fifth Avenue, New York, NY 10175 USA

Foreword

It is an honor and a pleasure to be asked to write the foreword for this useful book. When I was first shown *Counseling and Psychotherapy with College Students*, it was in the form of typed manuscript. I noticed immediately that virtually all of the chapter headings aroused my interest, since they cited problems and issues that clients seeking psychological help in university counseling centers are most likely to present. I read the book carefully and with deepening interest, often turning back to reexamine some intriguing piece of information and fix it in my mind.

This book will have a strong appeal for mental health practitioners who work with individuals struggling to master developmental problems of late adolescence and early adulthood. Consequently, health service-provider psychologists, social workers, psychiatrists, psychiatric nurses, counselors, and clergymen should find much of value in these pages.

It is written in a clear, easy-to-understand style. I found this an especially valuable aspect of the work because some of the subject matter is obviously complex. Specifically I refer to those chapters which deal with matters of central concern to the professional personnel employed in university and/or college settings: counseling the grieving student, the skillful use of brief psychotherapy by informed therapists in the context of a university-based counseling center, and the employment of imaging and early memory techniques for both diagnostic and treatment purposes. Developing professionals, along with those practitioners who have more experience, will find this material stimulating, and replete with useful information, including clearly explained techniques and case studies.

The grieving student is more frequently seen in counseling centers at the current time than we have realized. Unexpressed grief can be severely debilitating to the individual, with harmful effects on his or her social relationships and academic progress. Many times the student does not see the connection between a recent loss and the current problem.

The assessment of the grieving student, and subsequent grief therapy to help the individual through this stressful period, are discussed in a manner that makes explicit to the practitioner how to approach the problem, the nature of the constructive intervention, as well as to identify some of the modal fears that individuals who experience distorted grief reactions may share. Much of the relevant grief literature is pulled together in the presentation of this timely subject.

Today there are greater numbers of divorces than ever before, resulting in more broken homes and single parent families. Knowledge about counseling the student party to a broken marriage is a necessity for the mental health professional.

There are only a few training institutions in the country that have seriously studied the nature of brief psychotherapy and have conducted research on the subject. As one of these institutions, the Counseling and Psychological Services Center at Duke University is eminently well qualified to participate in this symposium. Brief psychotherapy is of great importance to counseling centers, which typically are not administratively organized to provide reconstructive therapy on a routine basis.

The chapter examines the qualities in the client that make brief therapy best suited for him or her. Universities usually go on the quarter or semester system, in accordance with which natural breaks occur several times per year; this situation makes brief therapy a more appropriate intervention in these settings, as the student's anticipations of times at which therapy can be expected to end are understood and accepted. The prerequisites a therapist needs if he or she wishes to practice this type of intervention are discussed in the chapter, as well.

Brief psychotherapy is not conceptualized here simply as a compression of long-term therapy; it is, rather, a distinct mode of intervention unto itself. Not only does this chapter deal with the personal makeups of both clients and therapists necessary to participating in brief therapy, but the tasks of the therapist are treated in a convincing manner, too.

At the end of this interesting unit, there is a summary of research studies on brief therapy which indicates that, for some clients with certain types of problems, it is the therapy of choice, and can be as effective as therapies of longer duration.

The book closes with a report of a study that was done by the Counseling and Psychological Services Center. In essence, the study "examined the commonly employed components of counseling in order to ascertain whether different groups of students respond to these components in different ways."

The research included three areas of investigation, but one area that had special importance for counseling centers dealt with clients' ratings of satisfaction with components of the counseling process, when the client population was broken down into the categories of sex, age, and numbers of sessions attended. Some interesting results gleaned from the large number that the study yielded were: encouragement by the therapist was more closely related to satisfaction for women than for men, whereas men responded to "warmth" by the therapist with higher satisfaction ratings. Men reported feeling "more understood" by the therapist than did women. The older the client, the more apt he or she was to indicate satisfaction with the counseling experience. Increased insight into problems was rated more satisfying to older students than to younger ones. The research seemed to investigate the practical sorts of problems about which counseling center personnel are often wondering.

Throughout the book, one senses that all the authors were writing with years of experience behind them. There is a frequent sharing of the subtle art/science of psychological intervention that cannot be acquired simply through a knowledge of the relevant literature, or conscientious scholarship.

I can only praise the care with which the central topics of this book were chosen. Almost without exception, the chapters focus upon major concerns of personnel employed in university counseling centers. The authors approach these topics with consistent vigor: Repeatedly, the reader is presented with a brief theoretical discussion of the subject; frequently this is followed by explanations of appropriate techniques and interventions, and then illustrated by short, relevant case examples--often no more than a paragraph long--and the point is clearly made.

I was intrigued with the discussion of self-psychology and object relations theory as treatment interventions applicable within the time constraints imposed by the administrative practicalities that influence counseling centers. Because this is my area of professional interest, I read these sections with increased attention and, perhaps, a more "critical eye." I found fresh, provocative insights in this chapter's treatment of the seminal work of Drs. Margaret Mahler and Heinz Kohut on separation-individuation and the solidification of the self, pointing up metaphorical parallels experienced by college students who are making the transition from adolescent status and dependence upon the parents, to young adulthood and further individuation.

The reader must be mindful throughout this book of the relatively large number of psychological issues discussed, as well as the intricacy of the theoretical positions that relate to them, and yet be grateful for the lucid, straightforwardness with which these issues are handled--it bespeaks a deep understanding of the particular areas and issues.

Handling the student who is so disturbed as to require psychiatric management receives careful attention. This broad topic is discussed comprehensively, with a heavy measure of common sense guiding the expertise and technical knowledge required in dealing with students who are experiencing emotional crises. The philosophy behind the judicious use of diagnostic labels applied to students in sensitively discussed, with the author pointing out occasions when inappropriate labeling may prove harmful by interfering with later treatment plans for the student.

In academic, institutional settings it is often both unwise and unrealistic to insinuate to the student that "everything" he or she says will be completely confidential, regardless of the situation. The author effectively clarifies instances in which other members of the institution with a "need to know" should properly be brought into the treatment planning for the student's best interest.

The topic of students who ultimately require medication for continued functioning within the university is nicely articulated here. The reader will find the proper methods of discussing proposed medication with students, and is advised of the possible consequences of uninformed counseling regarding this issue.

The study is well written in a down-to-earth, expository manner. Its subject matter, well organized both within the book and within individual chapters, follows a logical progression of topics that enhances its utility.

To me, the book seems essential for professionals in a large number of mental health settings, but especially so for college- or university-based mental health practitioners, who will find the wide spectrum of topics treated in an interesting manner of presentation both readable and relevant.

Paul T. King

Preface

"What specific method of treatment will work best with a particular person experiencing a certain type of problem?" is a question continually facing every practitioner. Focusing on the population of university students, this book gives detailed attention to the management of common presenting problems ranging from hospitalization to vocational counseling.

The volume begins with a thorough review of the salient literature pertaining to brief counseling and psychotherapy, especially with regard to students, by Dr. Rolffs Pinkerton, ABPP, Director of the Psychology Internship Program at Counseling and Psychological Services, Duke University. The chapter offers a discussion of student selection variables and necessary therapist functions.

Other topics include the psychotherapeutic treatment of the grieving student, the perfectionistic student, the student with disturbed self-esteem, and the student with psychosomatic problems. Research regarding the efficacy of utilizing early memories in the counseling process with students is presented. In the final chapter, the results of a study examining specific factors of the counseling/psychotherapy process that were found to be most helpful with certain subgroups of students are discussed. The students were categorized by age, sex, and number of sessions attended. This study employed pre- and post-treatment measures of anxiety and depression as well as post-treatment student satisfaction ratings. Various elements of treatment are correlated with the satisfaction ratings and comparisons between subgroups are made in order to ascertain which elements of counseling are perceived to be most therapeutic by each group.

The particular developmental issues of this age group are taken into account in considering the application of the various treatment methods that are presented for use with university students. Case illustrations are plentiful throughout the volume.

Acknowledgments

We are most appreciative of the excellent secretarial assistance given by Mrs. Sharon Jacobs and the superlative editorial assistance provided by Ms. Jean C. Hughes. For the collection and organization of our survey data, we express our gratitude to Mrs. Helen T. Biggers. We do wish to express our deep appreciation to Mr. William J. Griffith, Vice-President for Student Affairs at Duke University, for his continued encouragement and support of our work with students and related research conducted in the course of that work.

Joseph E. Talley

W. J. Kenneth Rockwell

Table of Contents

List of Tables

Counseling
and Psychotherapy
with College Students

Brief Individual Counseling and Psychotherapy with Students

Rolffs S. Pinkerton

BACKGROUND

The great majority of counseling and psychotherapy with college students is brief. The reasons for this are apparent: the usually acute and transient nature of the emotional and developmental crises occurring within the context of a relatively healthy ego, the students' high degree of motivation ("readiness") to embark on personal explorations, psychological mindedness, and the capacity to engage with another while at the same time wishing to preserve autonomy. Our counseling and mental health services are designed to accommodate these characteristics, minimize waiting lists, and, hopefully, meet students where they are. In conjunction with the cyclical nature of the academic calendar, these factors provide the essential ingredients for effective short-term treatment to take place.

Brief psychotherapy with students has been practiced since the time university mental health services began to appear in the United States. The interested reader is urged to note especially the contributions of Wedge (1958), Funkenstein (1959), and Farnsworth (1966). While early references to psychological interventions with the college population acknowledged the brevity of the number of sessions (Chassell 1940; Blos 1946; Gurman & Gordon 1948; and Gundle & Kraft 1956), it was only later that articles identified the service provided as "brief" or "short-term" (Faries 1955; Carlson 1958; Blaine 1957; Speers 1962; Whittington 1962; and Sifneos 1966). Interestingly, over the course of the past 25 years, little has changed regarding the nature of treatment, as the following comment by Wedge (1958) illustrates:

> *I find that somewhere between eight and twelve*
> *hours of therapy usually covers the total period*
> *of treatment . . . the reason therapy is so*
> *short is that immediately after one presents*
> *the patient with a challenge or shows surprise*
> *(and I mean surprise as an active interpretation),*
> *and he accepts this . . . he usually begins the*
> *most remarkable series . . . of explorations of*
> *other modes of behavior in his life [pp. 311-312].*

Since then brief counseling and psychotherapy has continued
to be the intervention of choice in the university setting
(Posin 1969; Binder & Weiskopf 1975; Hanfmann 1978; Podolnick
1979; Goodheart 1982; and Gelso & Johnson 1983a).

The intent of this chapter is to present an overview of
brief counseling and psychotherapy in the college counseling
and mental health service. It is based on our experience at
Duke University's Counseling and Psychological Services (CAPS)
as well as the clinical and empirical observations of others.

The theoretical orientation ascribed to at CAPS is based
on psychodynamic theory and is viewed within the framework of
young adult development. The assessment and subsequent understanding of the student is brought about through careful
determination of the precipitating element(s) leading the
individual to seek help, identifying the central conflict,
and discovering how it is maintained through psychological
defense mechanisms. The length of therapy is flexible and
may extend from one to approximately 20 sessions depending
on the degree of psychological impairment, the academic
calendar, and goals of treatment. The psychotherapeutic
intervention is eclectic and pragmatic. It involves problem
solving, environmental management, the teaching of coping
skills, suggestion, confrontation, interpretation, discussion
of the therapist-student relationship, and experiential
exercises, or a combination thereof. The setting is supportive and geared to promote trust, self-exploration and a
theraputic alliance in reaching treatment goals.

Short-term counseling and psychotherapy is not only
intrinsic to work with university students, the majority of
psychotherapeutic contacts in the general population are time
limited, whether initially planned as such or not (Butcher &
Koss 1978). An often quoted survey by the National Center
for Health Statistics of 979,000 patients seen in some form
of psychiatric treatment from July 1963 to June 1964 found the
average number of visits to be 4.7 (1966). These findings
are, in general, consistent with other studies indicating a
substantial percent of patients conclude psychotherapy within
the first six to eight sessions. Garfield's (1978) review of
research pertaining to continuation in psychotherapy reveals
that most patients terminate at about the sixth interview.

It is of interest to note that fewer than 10 percent continue
for 15 or more sessions, 25 being a number still well within
the limits described for brief psychotherapy (Alexander &
French 1946; Malan 1976; Marmor 1979; Strupp & Hadley 1979;
Davanloo 1980; and Wolberg 1980). These data are further
supported by Lorian (1974) and Bloom (1981). The last inves-
tigator noted that the expectation of the patient is that
significant improvement should come within five sessions and
recovery from complaints within ten. This confirms the
results of a survey by Garfield and Wolpin (1963) that found
that 70 percent of those being served at outpatient clinics
expected to receive ten or fewer sessions.

In college counseling and mental health services brief
trends are also evident. Dorosin and associates (1976) note
that the number of students seen three or fewer times at the
Stanford University Mental Health Service is approximately
50 to 60 percent. Haggerty and colleagues (1980) at the
University of North Carolina, Chapel Hill, report a similar
finding, 57 percent making three or fewer contacts. At
Counseling and Psychological Services, Duke University, our
annual statistics present a similar picture. During the
academic year 1982-83, of those students coming for psychosocial intervention, 50 percent were seen once or twice, 75
percent for six or fewer visits, and 90 percent for 13 sessions or less. Similarly, at the Rutgers College Counseling
Center 89 percent of students continuing after the initial
intake evaluation were treated in 12 sessions or less (Goodheart 1982). Friedman and Coons (1969) reported a mean
number of three visits in their survey of 647 new patients
seen at the Psychiatric Division of the Indiana University
Student Health Center during the 1966-67 academic calendar.
These findings are largely in concert with earlier surveys.
In *Mental Health on the Campuses--A Field Study*, Glasscote
and Fishman (1973) reported the experience of four separate
college counseling programs in which those students seen
three or less times, expressed as a percentage of all students served was 60 percent, 44 percent, 48 percent, and 60
percent. These figures appear somewhat lower than those of
a more recent large-scale survey conducted by Dunn and
associates (1980). Collecting data during the 1975-76, 1976-
77 academic years at the College Center, a comprehensive
mental health facility serving students in the Greater Boston
area, the authors determined that the mean number of visits
for all students seen (814) was 8.1. What makes this survey
especially significant is the heterogeneous group of schools
(and students) served including universities, professional
programs, schools of performing arts, and hospital-based
schools of nursing and health.

By way of summary, therefore, it is evident that the vast
majority of college students availing themselves of university

counseling and mental health services are seen for brief
psychotherapy and that a substantial portion are served for
very brief periods.

IS BRIEF COUNSELING AND PSYCHOTHERAPY
COMPATIBLE WITH STUDENTS?

Recognizing that most psychotherapy with students is
brief, we can begin to speculate as to the reasons. Factors
we have considered, while not exhaustive, include: (1) the
need for autonomy and control; (2) motivation for and expectation of treatment; (3) the nature of developmental crises;
and (4) general satisfaction with a brief number of encounters.

Many college students are immersed in a struggle to
manage their dependent and independent strivings. The desire
for autonomy and control is often countered equally by the
need for direction and safety provided by important persons
in the social surroundings. By the fact that it is initiated
through an awareness of having a problem and due to the
necessity of having to make an appointment to see a professional (in which there is at least the implication that one
will be advised and directed), psychotherapy energizes the
young adult to avoid a prolonged encounter and to move as
hastily as possible toward resolution. If a successful
series of sessions has taken place, such movement does indeed
leave the student with a more positive sense of self-worth
and mastery, notably with regard to her/his coping abilities.

Students observed coming to our service are motivated
to resolve their difficulties and to do so in rapid fashion.
Hopefully, this "set" is in accord with the views of the
therapist whose goal is to work within the students' time
frame as well as to avoid building a waiting list. It is
notable in this regard that a significant number of college
counseling and mental health services delimit the number of
visits (generally 8 to 12). Students are made aware of this
prior to or after coming in for their initial appointment.
Thus, their energy is channeled to work successfully within
a time-limited mode. This observation is consistent with the
conclusions drawn by Gelso and Johnson in their studies (1983b)
that students did not expect counseling of long duration
and, in fact, assumed they would receive significantly fewer
than 12 sessions. Finally, this arrangement fits well into
the academic calendar as do other activities in the student's
life. The semester cycle provides a natural beginning and
ending for the therapy experience.

The period of young adulthood is a time of continuing
personality change and adaptation. Leaving home, beginning
the process of gaining autonomy and relinquishing dependency

ties to kith and kin, learning to balance one's personal needs with those of a new social structure and with those in authority, defining and redefining values, and accommodating varying forms of intimacy are some of the potential crises-producing maturational milestones in the lives of university students. Difficulties centering around these issues are often brought to our attention in counseling and mental health services. The fact that these crises are acute and that the motivation to overcome them is great coupled with their generally transient nature make such presenting problems most amenable to brief therapy.

Our experience and that of others (Dorosin et al. 1976 and Haggerty et al. 1980), reveal that a significant percentage of students seen in brief treatment, even with *very* brief interventions (one to three sessions), report satisfaction with their experience. This will be elaborated upon in more detail in a later section of this chapter. For now, it is considered only for the implications it offers regarding the compatibility of brief therapy for the student.

Does this imply that *all* students are satisfied with a brief modality of treatment? Obviously, the answer is "no." As will be noted in the next section regarding selection variables, a portion of students can be served most appropriately in long-term therapy, particularly those with significant ego disruption and/or those requiring reconstruction of the personality. Even those students, however, who are determined (by the therapist) to be a candidate for brief treatment may be dissatisfied as the following response to one of our CAPS satisfaction survey questionnaires reveals: "Actually, I was not really helped--each time I began to pull myself together I was told I didn't really need to come anymore. I usually felt more lost than otherwise after a couple of sessions." The lack of empathy on the part of the therapist is evidenced by this response and underscores the need for a careful assessment and an equally thorough review of what the student is asking for and what is needed. Not withstanding this and some similar examples, however, our observation is that by and large the opportunity to engage in brief treatment is compatible with the expectations of the great majority of students we serve.

STUDENT SELECTION VARIABLES

The characteristics generally considered predictive of successful brief psychotherapy with college students are also those recognized as associated with successful brief psychotherapy in general. A number of writers have elaborated on these dimensions, most notably, Sifneos (1972), Mann (1973), Malan (1976), Marmor (1979), Davanloo (1980), and Mann and Goldman (1982).

The student has often been referred to as the "ideal" psychotherapy patient. This is largely due to the fact that many of the prerequisites for success in college are also variables considered to be important for success in brief therapy. It is without surprise, therefore, that we are typically presented with bright, articulate, intrapersonally curious people who have already developed the ability to relate with some degree of comfort with another person. In a recent investigation conducted at the University Counseling Center, University of Maryland, Adelstein et al. (1983) attempted to identify developments that emerge in the client and the treatment situation in time-limited therapy that are predictors of continued growth when treatment ends. The authors conclude that three developments, in combination, seem most predictive. These include client insight, communication skills, and improved self-concept. Considered together, these factors seem to lead to long-term change. Thus, when their clients began to develop appropriately and positively in regard to how they viewed themselves, started exhibiting insight, and expressed themselves more effectively with others, the chances were greater that therapeutic changes would remain durable. By contrast, maintaining a central focus, a characteristic underscored by many writers, was found to be unrelated to lasting change effects.

Notwithstanding the limited research on this topic, a number of characteristics can now be considered that augur well for successful outcome in brief psychotherapy.

Motivation

This variable received considerable attention in the works of Malan (1963, 1976), Sifneos (1968, 1971, 1972), and most recently Keithly et al. (1980) and Strupp (1980a, 1980b, 1980c). On the basis of years of clinical experience Sifneos (1980) was led to delineate seven criteria which he considered valuable as predictive of successful outcome in a Short-Term Anxiety-Provoking Psychotherapy. These include: (1) the ability to recognize that the symptoms are psychological in nature; (2) an ability to give an honest and truthful account of one's psychological difficulties; (3) a willingness to participate actively in the therapy; (4) curiosity, introspection, and ability to understand oneself; (5) a willingness to explore and to experiment; (6) realistic expectations of the results of psychotherapy; (7) a willingness to make a tangible sacrifice. Because of Sifneos' extensive experience in working with college youth, attention to this aspect of student selection is especially important.

With most university students motivation in therapy is generally high, in concert with their attitudes toward academic and vocational endeavors and interpersonal dealings. Nevertheless, this is not to say that all college students

are motivated for psychotherapy. Those administratively
directed to the service, often due to episodes of acting out,
as well as those urged by parents, often in order to meet
parents' needs, appear less likely to succeed. The hallmark
of motivation is evident in the student who recognizes a
psychologically destructive element within, expresses curiosity as to its origins and nature, and is desirous of learning
about it and finding a reasonably compatible way of dealing
with it.

Relatively Healthy Ego

A number of investigators underscore the importance of
working with students who have intact egos. Keilson et al.
(1979) expressed doubt whether time-limited therapy should
be considered for the most disturbed clients and recommended
that research be devoted toward devising time-limited approaches that might be effective with such clients. Along
a similar line Gelso et al. (1983) related:

> For the more disturbed client, we cannot currently
> recommend time-limited therapy. . . . If an agency
> deems it important to abbreviate treatment duration
> because clients must wait too long for treatment
> when it is open ended, then time-limited therapy
> with the more disturbed client might best be viewed
> as either crisis oriented or preparatory to refer-
> ral and long-term treatment [p. 58].

In their summary of a series of investigations recently concluded at the University of Maryland Counseling Service,
Gelso and Johnson (1983b) pointed out that clients who viewed
themselves as less troubled, who had been troubled for a
shorter time period, and who came to their counseling in a
high state of readiness to change and were perceived by their
therapist as being effective in relating, appeared to be the
best candidates for time-limited therapy. Dunn et al. (1980)
observed that students who were given more serious diagnoses
at the College Center in Boston were seen longer in psychotherapy than those with less serious diagnoses.

These investigations support what has long been considered important by experienced clinicians--namely, evidence
of intelligence and educational achievement, the ability to
assume responsibility, having had at least one meaningful
relationship in the past and hence the capacity to establish
trust, and the ability to relate to the therapist initially
in therapy.

Psychological Mindedness and the Willingness
to Accept Interpretation

The quality of examining oneself with a reasonable degree
of openness, while at the same time allowing the therapist
to offer interpretations, is not an altogether easy task given
the proclivity of most young adults to retain their autonomous and independent thinking. This characteristic is particularly significant when doing insight work. Hence, the
student must enter therapy with some willingness to accept
authority and the therapist's formulations, observations, and
suggestions. We noted this to be especially valuable in very
brief interventions of one or two sessions (Pinkerton & Rockwell 1982).

The Ability to Establish a Rapid and Positive
Relationship with the Therapist

Unlike the gradual development of the therapeutic alliance in long-term psychotherapy, it is imperative in brief
work that the student "connect" rapidly and positively with
the therapist. In a well-controlled outcome study conducted
as a part of the Vanderbilt Psychotherapy Research Project,
Strupp and Hadley (1979) investigated specific vs. nonspecific
factors in the brief individual psychotherapy performed by
experienced psychotherapists with 15 male students (17 to 24
years old) suffering from relatively mild neurotic and characterological disturbances. A comparable group was treated
by college professors chosen specifically for their ability
to form understanding relationships. There were no differences as to the quality of outcome between those two groups
(both improved on a wide range of outcome and process measures) and both treated groups exceeded the controls. In
interpreting the results, the authors offered the following
conclusions: (1) regardless of who was providing the treatment (experienced therapists or college professors) positive
results appeared to be attributable to the healing effects of
a benign relationship, (2) therapeutic change seemed to occur
more readily if the patient was capable of taking advantage
of the relationship (low resistance and high motivation) and
the therapist was experienced (by the patient) as being caring and maintaining genuine interest, and (3) while the technique of professional therapists did not seem to result in
measurably superior results, they did appear to advance the
healing process within a good personal relationship.

Factors Contraindicating Brief
Counseling and Psychotherapy

A relatively small proportion of students present to the
college counseling mental health service with accompanying
severe psychopathology. It is not expected that students
manifesting psychotic episodes, major depressions (unipolar
or bipolar), or a borderline personality organization will
have the ego resources available to benefit from short-term
treatment. The therapist needs to be especially mindful of
this and be in a position to make a rapid and accurate diagnostic assessment. With such students the therapist should
have ready access to long-term therapy referral sources. If
not, the therapist must be prepared to enter into an extended,
time-unlimited contract. To leave the job otherwise incom-
plete will only disappoint and frustrate the student, leaving
a sense of distrust of the psychotherapeutic process and the
added feelings of futility and rejection.

THERAPIST SELECTION VARIABLES

It is not expected that all therapists will be effective
at brief counseling and psychotherapy with students. There
are those who do not see its value or, if they do, do not
consider themselves qualified or willing to pursue it. Further, there are those who, for whatever reason, do not enjoy
working with young adults. Because therapist variables are
inextricably bound to technique and approach, this section
will address those *personal* qualities that appear to fit comfortably with doing brief treatment in the college setting.

Belief in the Effectiveness of Brief Counseling
and Psychotherapy with Young Adults

There is good clinical documentation as well as recent
empirical justification to underscore the value of the therapist's belief in the worth of brief therapy. Gelso et al.
(1983), summarizing their research on factors influencing
outcome in time-limited therapy noted: "therapists' confidence that the treatment they could offer would be helpful
. . . and expected enjoyment in working with the client were
especially associated with . . . outcomes" (p. 112).

Comfort with the Position of Authority

Brief counseling and psychotherapy will be facilitated
if the therapist is comfortable with the position of author-

ity and is willing to speak with confidence about findings
and formulations early in therapy while acknowledging to the
student that they are preliminary and are based on hypotheses
and are open to questioning. It is important to underscore
that care should be given not to relate in an authoritarian
manner which only promotes resistance. Rather, formulations
can be presented as tentative and preliminary and with the
consideration that they may or may not fit with how the student is seeing the situation.

Comfort with Modest Goals

In keeping with setting limited objectives for treatment,
the therapist must also feel relatively comfortable with the
goal(s) agreed upon. Being able to conclude work with the
student while at the same time wondering if what has been set
in motion will continue to unfold is not an easy task. Certainly the therapist who is seeking the "complete cure" will
be most incompatible with the process of doing brief work.

Ability to Come to a Rapid and
Accurate Assessment

This involves at least two stages of activity. First,
the therapist must recognize the degree of psychopathology
present (if any) and come to a determination regarding
whether the student should be referred for long-term treatment or if there is sufficient ego strength and resilience
to work within a brief time frame. This process might best
be understood as an initial screening evaluation. Being
satisfied at this level of the assessment, the therapist is
then in the position to more clearly determine the problem.
The value of isolating a central or focal conflict has been
underscored as being of particular importance (Sifneos 1972;
Mann 1973; Marmor 1979; Davanloo 1980).

Ability to Rapidly Establish
a Positive Relationship

Our experience suggests that this is a crucial aspect of
therapist selection for work with college students. Research
supports this clinical impression for the general population.
Malan (1963) noted that therapists who reflect enthusiasm in
their work enhance the therapeutic relationship as well as
the outcome. Nash et al. (1965) found that therapists who
were judged to have offered the best therapeutic relationship
produced more positive outcomes. Similarly, Frank (1974),

reviewing a 25 year progress report of research on therapeutic components in psychotherapy, underscored the importance of the quality of the interaction between therapist and patient and the fact that it serves as a major criterion for success in brief psychotherapy.

THERAPIST FUNCTIONS IN BRIEF COUNSELING
AND PSYCHOTHERAPY WITH STUDENTS

Put in its simplest form, the therapist does what she/he can to direct the treatment at a pace, and in a direction that meets the goals ascribed, in the briefest time possible. While our objective is a modest one, it hopes at the least to "set a process in motion" that can be sustained upon termination. This assumes, of course, that a careful and thorough assessment has been made of the presenting problem and that the student has been evaluated as suitable for brief treatment. The following considerations culled from the literature are confirmed by our own experience.

Assist the Student in Defining
the Nature of the Problem

While most college students are generally aware of the event(s) that bring them to the service, some are not. For example, a young man presented with symptoms of depression. Only during the initial contact did he determine that his feelings of dysphoria had come about since the graduation of his two closest companions. He seemed surprised by this revelation and while there was more to the picture than this connection, the knowledge of it seemed to give him an initial sense of relief. Socarides (1954), writing on the usefulness of extremely brief psychoanalytic contacts referred to this technique as "spotlighting" for the patient conflicts previously out of conscious awareness.

Shortly, within one or two sessions, the therapist interprets to the student what is believed to be the core problem or conflict. A freshman student presented with a crisis involving homesickness. Being psychologically close to but geographically distant from his parents he found his adjustment to college most troublesome. As we soon discovered, the framework for his feelings was a strong dependence on his mother and father who, in turn, reinforced their son's need for them. When the student was alerted to the nature of the association with them he began to view his situation differently. He was able to identify his desire, on the one hand, to establish his autonomy but also his coexisting need to remain dependent. The student was well endowed with ego strength and had, in fact, partly chosen to attend an out-of-state institution in order to "get away." Within a few weeks he launched further into his academic pursuits, joined a university organization and began to reach out to others.

Maintain a Focus

While there has been some recent research that contradicts the notion that a focus must be maintained in successful brief counseling and psychotherapy (Adelstein et al. 1983), the overwhelming consensus from clinical observation is that this is a most important element of brief treatment (Wolberg 1965; Sifneos 1972; Marmor 1979; and Davanloo 1980). Our observations support the consensus. While the therapist does not need to handle this in a rigid and controlling manner, a sensitive and gentle moving in a direction to fulfill the goal of treatment is essential. It is assumed as well that the therapist engage the student *actively*. We have discovered, as have others, that long silences do not augur well for brief treatment with the young adult.

Encourage Ventilation

This function requires no elaboration. A principal element outlined in all approaches to brief treatment is the value of encouraging the expression of emotion on the part of the patient. This is no less true of the college student.

Promoting Insight

Several years ago Menninger and Holzman (1973) outlined their now familiar "triangle of insight" in which they underscored the value of patients learning about the nature of their conflict(s) as they are presented in (1) their current relationships with important others, (2) significant figures in the past such as parents and siblings, and (3) the relationship with the therapist. Davanloo (1980) and Marmor (1979) have since then underscored the value of this approach in short-term dynamic psychotherapy and Love and Widen (1982) have successfully applied it to work with college students. The following case from our Service illustrates this function. A sophomore woman presented herself due to experiencing feelings of worthlessness and depression following a recent breakup with her boyfriend. After much ventilation of her feelings during the initial several sessions it became apparent that she also wanted to avoid such a catastrophe in the future and was curious whether there may have been elements in her behavior that had led to the dissolution of the association with her boyfriend. As her story unfolded it became clear that she had maintained a deferential, subservient attitude toward him. Her position was to please at all cost. What in fact had partially contributed to the breakup was her boyfriend's desire to date other women. While the student was clearly uncomfortable with this, in characteristic fashion she chose to go along with it "because it was what I felt he wanted." In subsequent sessions multiple examples of this interpersonal style emerged as revealed in a review of her previous relationships, notably her earlier association with her parents. Throughout this time the student remained ambivalent, as well, regarding her appointments at the service. While initially appearing to be resistant, it became more obvious that she did not feel worthy of the time she took up in therapy and was concerned that she was being a burden. As her level of self-awareness grew she resolved to take better care of herself, most notably by affirming her worth and relinquishing her self-demeaning position in relationship to others. Her treatment ended shortly thereafter and, in order to adopt skills to assist her growth, she subsequently entered an assertiveness training group.

A RECENT CONSIDERATION: VERY BRIEF INTERVENTION
AND PSYCHOTHERAPY WITH STUDENTS

Several years ago our staff became curious to discover the frequency with which students came to the service for only one or two appointments. We asked ourselves if they were feeling disappointed with the intervention provided or were we not "connecting." While these concerns touched us we were also aware that, by and large, those students seen so briefly were reporting at the end of one or two interviews that they were satisfied. Moreover, when reached by telephone several months later, these same students typically recalled their contact(s) clearly and offered comments indicative of its subsequent value to them. We began to study this phenomenon more closely and were gratified to find that a rather substantial literature on one or two session psychotherapy was available with respect to the general psychiatric population (Rockwell & Pinkerton 1982) as well as several studies of very brief contacts in university settings (Ichikawa 1961; Spears 1962; Dorosin et al. 1976; Hanfmann 1979; and Haggerty et al. 1980). Such therapy has been variously referred to as VBI (very brief intervention) by Dorosin et al. (1976) and Haggerty et al. (1980), productive brief encounters by Hanfmann (1979), and one or two session psychotherapy by Pinkerton and Rockwell (1982). The number of sessions varies from one to four and although one could debate the merits of one versus four sessions or, for that matter, how these numbers substantially differ from five or six, suffice it to say that for a substantial number of students, very brief therapy seems to fulfill treatment needs. In examining this form of therapy in more detail, notably as it pertains to our population at Duke University, the following applications appear most evident.

Reviewing and Approving Psychological Work Already Done and/or Affirming a Psychological Decision Already Made

A 20-year-old junior presented herself to the service in a mild state of anxiety precipitated by a letter she had received from her hometown boyfriend the previous week. She reported that the two had been steadily seeing each other for a year and a half and within recent months her boyfriend had been pursuing her with the intent of getting married. While she acknowledged they had discussed this possibility previously, the conclusion they had reached was that she should first graduate from college. It was thus with some surprise and anger that she received his most recent correspondence. In it he again argued for a commitment for an earlier marriage and his concluding comments had taken on a more threatening tone, namely, if they could not make such an arrangement then perhaps the relationship should be dissolved. The student had been bewildered and somewhat frightened by his position. She spoke of her love for him but at the same time was clearly committed to maintaining her stand for an after-graduation wedding. While she felt reasonably good about her decision she wanted specifically to "get an objective opinion to see if 'I'm doing this right.'" The therapist listened supportively. In the end it was stated that, given the background she had presented as well as the feelings she was experiencing about the matter, her decision seemed sound. She stated that she felt considerable relief after hearing this and acknowledged that it was "good to know I'm on the right track." The student left feeling satisfied with this one contact.

Clarifying a Diagnostic Concern

We have discovered that a small portion of students come to our service with a problem concerning whether their emotional and/or behavioral reactions are "normal." Given the fact that what constitutes normality or abnormality is difficult to define, anxiety about this issue can become quite ego-disrupting for the student. There are a variety of examples that illustrate this point: the student who (1) questions the appropriateness of a grief reaction to the loss of a loved one, (2) has doubts about sexual identity because of having thus far chosen to preserve virginity until marriage or at least until a committed partner is available, (3) chooses not to drink alcohol or to drink in moderation when "everyone else is getting smashed," (4) makes a career decision which is not in keeping with family expectations. These are but a few examples of issues brought to our attention that imply directly or indirectly that the student has concerns about being "different" and is in need of some external verification that the chosen approach to the situation is not the product of mental disorder. Our experience has been that when the therapist encounters a situation of this kind, and indeed no psychopathology is evident, the therapist should state explicitly that the student's mental health appears to be in good order. A positive statement based on a clear understanding of the problem can be very ego-supportive for the student.

Environmental Stress Management

Students will frequently seek out the counseling and mental health service in the hope of relieving an external stressor, whether they are initially aware of this fact or not. This will sound most familiar to those who have assisted anxious students in obtaining a course drop, postponing an exam, or finding ways to manage tension and anxiety. An 18-year-old freshman appeared at our service subsequent to recurrent panic attacks he was having in preparing for a final examination in physics. He had been an A+ student in high school but found his first semester of college most rigorous. Although he presented as an obsessive young man with high achievement needs, it was clear following initial exploration that he had no interest in changing this aspect of his personality. His immediate concern was to relieve his present state of distress. Following a brief historical review, it was discovered that he felt most calm and was able to do his best studying in a quiet and relatively peaceful atmosphere. This he had been unable to experience in his dorm room or the library in recent days. Given this information the therapist recommended that he spend several nights in the infirmary. The student agreed and arrangements were subsequently made. He returned three days later looking rested, significantly more relaxed, and reporting optimism regarding his upcoming examination. He was seen for these two visits only and, while acknowledging appreciation for the service provided, he felt no need to return for further appointments. In addition to demonstrating a positive result of environmental manipulation, this case illustrates as well the value of working with stu-

dents at the point of their expressed need. While it can be
argued that the student would be likely to continue to experience difficulties with academic demands until such time as
he gained insight into his obsessional achieving nature, it
can likewise be stated that efforts to move him in that direction would most likely have proven futile. The student evi-
dently felt positive about his experience with the service
We conjecture that brief positive experiences help to enable
some students to seek more extensive therapy (even years)
later.

The cases presented are generally in keeping with those
principles of management used in crisis intervention advanced
by Caplan (1964). In each case the therapeutic goal was to
reestablish the student's equilibrium and to assist in the
development of a greater sense of mastery than experienced at
the time the appointment was made. While it is apparent that
no effort was made to foster insight (it is important to note
that in each case the student was not asking for this), it is
believed that resolution of their crises did have an ego-
enhancing effect.

Promoting Insight

Perhaps the most rewarding work in very brief therapy is
that which leads to insight and greater personal awareness on
the part of the student. A 23-year-old graduate student came
to the service stating that she had been feeling increasingly
irritable over the course of the past several weeks. She found
it difficult to concentrate and acknowledged that her appetite
had sleep had been poor. She then recounted that during the
previous Christmas vacation, a close male friend had been killed
in an automobile accident. She described her friend as having
"lived on the wild side." He was characterized as charming and
fun to be with but as having a reputation for recklessness and
irresponsibility. He was known to drink heavily and it was understood by members of the community that this likely led to his
accident and death. She registered confusion as to her feelings. At the time he died she was grief-stricken and recognized
it. She and friends talked openly as did she and her parents.
Although she continued to feel sadness and a sense of loss, she
nevertheless wondered if there might be something else troubling
her. She then talked of her previous association with her
friend. They had known each other for several years and she
commented on the fact that she "had known about his ways from
the time we met." Following this she asked the therapist if he
knew how people like that could change. Would psychotherapy be
of any help? The therapist was curious about her question and
wondered openly whether she was puzzled about what she could
have done to prevent the accident. She smiled knowingly and
related, "the thought had crossed my mind."

The second session began with the student stating that she had contemplated further whether she might have acted in some way to assist her friend. She went on to say that, having been aware of his impulsive behavior perhaps she could have done something. She then recalled that she had often been tempted to talk to him, point out his potentially de-structive behavior, but failed to do so out of fear that he would take unkindly to her criticism. At this point it appeared clear to the therapist that the source of her dis-comfort was less related to the sense of loss she experienced than her feeling of responsibility for her friend's death. She then told the story of a girlfriend of hers in the ninth grade. The account was similar. The friend became involved with drugs at an early age and ultimately became increasingly self-destructive. She began acting out sexually and finally got into difficulty with the law and later entered a deten-tion home. The student said that she had forgotten this event until now. She then spoke in an impassioned way about her sense of guilt. She proceeded to point out that she had been raised to be "her brother's keeper" and felt somehow that she had failed at this task. She related that she must have obtained this characteristic "honestly." Her parents had repeatedly made a point of emphasizing the value of loyalty to friends and regularly provided for the needs of others themselves. We connected the two events involving her friends and the therapist underscored his perception of her heightened sense of responsibility with its derivative of guilt.

There was a two-week hiatus before she returned for her third appointment. She came in reporting having had an especially good two weeks. She had been able to concentrate and she was now sleeping more regularly. We explored further how she had been raised and reviewed again the early admoni-tion to be responsible. She had thought more about our dis-cussions and had come to recognize numerous examples of how she had taken care of people. Another follow-up appointment was made. She was seen at that time for about fifteen min-utes during which it was clear that she was continuing to feel well and satisfied.

HOW EFFECTIVE IS BRIEF COUNSELING AND PSYCHOTHERAPY WITH STUDENTS?

At first glance it would appear that the college counsel-ing and mental health service lends itself well to research in brief psychotherapy, particularly when we consider the ready access to a contained, homogeneous, and bright (hence, easily measurable) population. Such has not been the case, however, and surprisingly little research is evident. Arn-

stein (1979), addressing the troubling problem of assessment
in psychotherapy at the Yale Mental Hygiene Clinic notes a
number of factors that hamper the researcher: (1) resistance
to completing protocols by an already overworked staff, (2)
difficulty in interpreting a high success rate because of
"transference" effects, (3) whether to use therapist opinion
or consumer satisfaction, (4) how to control for initial
severity or chronicity, and (5) how to define clear-cut variables, such as symptoms, patterns of emotional response, and
levels of functioning. These factors need to be considered
as well as the fact that the typical college counseling and
mental health service is not set up with research as a principal objective. Instead, our programs are identified as service units that may provide a training component. Research
generally takes a tertiary position, time allocated being
minimal due to direct service needs. This state of priorities is correspondingly reflected in budget allocations and
staffing and hiring practices. The result is that we find
ourselves in a catch-22 circumstance: In order for colleges
and universities to justify what has become a relatively
expensive operation, counseling and mental health services
staffs find it essential to produce evidence of the effectiveness of their work. This, in turn, requires time, money, and
available personnel.

Notwithstanding the above, the problem of determining the
quality of brief counseling and psychotherapy with college
students (even under more ideal research-producing conditions)
is reflected as well in the general state of the art of
assessment of short-term treatment in general. Butcher and
Koss (1978) in their excellent review of research on time-
limited and crisis-oriented interventions write:

> The research on outcome of brief psychotherapy
> has been plagued with difficulty. . . . One of
> the main problems with existing outcome studies
> involves the failure to utilize clear control
> groups and not specify the actual procedures used
> in brief therapy or crisis intervention [pp. 759-
> 760].

Research determining the value of brief counseling and
psychotherapy with college students can be grouped into two
categories: (1) outcome studies and (2) individual case
studies.

Outcome Research

Client satisfaction. The most popular method of determining the impact of brief counseling and psychotherapy has

been client satisfaction. Nigl and Weiss (1976), in a study designed to investigate therapist orientation and its effect on students' symptoms, discovered that regardless of the therapists' treatment approach, students rated themselves "healthier" one year after treatment than when they initially sought help at the mental health service. In a study designed to investigate the influence of time-limited therapy at the Counseling Service, University of Maryland, Keilson et al. (1979) investigated a sample of 42 clients representing the normal, moderately neurotic range of adjustment. Using the Index of Adjustment and Values (IAV) as the criterion measure, the authors compared outcomes of students receiving eight session time-limited therapy with those receiving open-ended therapy and those in a no-treatment control group. The results led the authors to conclude that time-limited therapy is a viable treatment for clients who are not seriously disturbed. Moreover, time-limited therapy seemed to produce as much change as open-ended treatment and the change was lasting. Weber and Tilley (1981) surveyed the attitudes of 207 students seen during a two-year period at the mental health service at the Medical College of Virginia. One hundred fifty-one (74 percent) completed a questionnaire designed to assess students' evaluation of services. Six months following the initial visit, 81 percent indicated they were feeling better, 12 percent felt the same, and 7 percent indicated they were feeling worse. Two-thirds of the students responding added positive comments on the evaluation questionnaire.

As mentioned previously, Dorosin et al. (1976) have identified a significant treatment phenomenon--the Very Brief Intervention (VBI). These investigators mailed satisfaction questionnaires to 220 students who had received mental health services at the Stanford University Clinic. This group included those who had been seen three or fewer times. Of the 54 percent who responded, 80 percent or more reported that they had had a positive experience. In this regard, 54 felt the contact had been "very helpful," and 41 described the experience as "moderately helpful." This investigation was later replicated at the University of North Carolina, Chapel Hill by Haggerty et al. (1980). The authors mailed the same questionnaire employed in the Stanford University study to 215 students seen three or fewer times. Although the return rate was only 40 percent, 72 percent of the respondents reported satisfaction with their treatment. In a survey done by Duke University's Counseling and Psychological Services (Chapter Nine), 150 satisfaction questionnaires were sent to a random sample of students seen for psychosocial reasons during the fall semester, 1981. Of the 67 percent (N = 81) who responded, 41 (65 percent) were seen for one to three visits. Confirming the studies done at Stanford and the University of North Carolina, our investigation revealed that students were satisfied with the services they received in one, two, or three visits.

Therapist ratings. Utilizing therapist ratings to determine brief psychotherapy outcome with 25 students at the Mental Health Division of the University of Massachusetts Health Services, Sarnat (1979) documented the following breakdown of outcome: (1) 42 percent improved functioning in the problem area, (2) 64 percent improved comfort in the problem area, (3) 82 percent global rating of treatment as "successful" and (4) 20 percent determined as having experienced growth in other areas.

Client satisfaction and therapist ratings. In an early outcome study, Allen and Janowitz (1964) surveyed 494 students seen for treatment at the University of Massachusetts. Approximately one-half responded. Of those, 26 percent felt genuinely helped, 29 percent said they had gained some insight and understanding but that their problem persisted to some extent, and 18 percent "got some ideas" from their visit(s) but went on to solve their own problems. When therapists rated the outcome of *all* 494 students seen, 43 percent emerged as improved. Using a self-report inventory and therapist chart notations, Brown et al. (1980) studied 242 students seen at the college mental health service at the University of Arizona. Self-rated improvement on major symptoms ranged from 81.8 percent to 88.4 percent for students receiving a diagnosis of anxiety neurosis, depressive neurosis, and adjustment reaction. By contrast, those with a diagnosis of personality disorder reported a 54.5 percent improvement. Therapist-rated improvement reflected in chart notations was uniformly lower (36.4 to 77.3 percent). Poey (1981) described the outcome of 32 students who were treated in between 4 and 15 sessions at the University of Massachusetts Mental Health Service. Questionnaires were administered to clients only prior to the initial session and to clients and therapists following the first and final sessions. Using a Likert-type rating scale as the criterion measure, results of the study supported the efficacy of brief therapy in reducing clients' target symptoms, discomfort/distress and interference with functioning levels. Unfortunately, this study was hampered because a substantial number of the original pool was lost due to early dropout and to being referred for long-term treatment.

Individual Case Studies

The individual case study offers the advantage of providing an in-depth analysis of one or several cases by means of a variety of process and outcome measures. In a relatively early case study analysis, Jacobs et al. (1968) evaluated the effectiveness of brief psychotherapy with three students. All were seen over a six-month period, two for 24 sessions and one for 16 sessions. Manifest distress and distortions in styles of adaptation (ego strength) were used as indexes of change. The authors employed weekly measures of manifest distress utilizing self-rating scales and therapist and judges' ratings of the patients' maladaptation. Ego strength was also assessed weekly over the course of treatment with independent judgments based on ratings of transcripts from sessions. The following results are summarized by the authors. Case A, 20-year-old female, improved significantly both in reduction of manifest symptomatology as well as in certain aspects of ego strength. Case B, 21-year-old male, was basically unchanged following the six months of treatment. It was determined that his ability to deal effectively with his impulses, self-image, capacity to manage frustration, and ability to function independently were at the same levels of disturbance at the second phase of treatment than they were in the first. It was determined, however, that he was better able to get along with others, a significant factor in that this had been his presenting complaint. Finally, Case C, 20-year-old female (seen 16 times), was regarded as the healthiest of the cases reported. She felt improvement in manifest distress over the course of treatment although the therapist and judges did not interpret a significant change. Regarding ego-strength ratings, the student was more able to assert herself and slightly more able to maintain a positive self-concept without continued reinforcement from others. Frustration tolerance, on the other hand, did not improve and remained a problem for her.

In an attempt to discover those variables which influence success and failure in time-limited psychotherapy, Strupp (1980a, 1980b, 1980c) has conducted a series of investigations as a part of the Vanderbilt Psychotherapy Research Project. These investigations are especially relevant for work with students because of the systematic outcome and process measures used and the detailed study of complete process recordings. All investigations involved highly experienced professional psychotherapists. Each treated his or her patients in individual time-limited psychotherapy (up to 25 hours in twice-a-week sessions). The students were single males and all were enrolled at Vanderbilt University at the time the studies were conducted. Their ages ranged from 18 to 25; all suffered from anxiety, depression, and difficulties in relating to peers, notably the opposite sex.

Results of these investigations led Strupp to offer the following conclusions:

1. Given a therapist who is basically empathic and benign, the principal determinants of a successful psychotherapeutic outcome are traceable to the student.

2. If the above conditions exist and if the student's past life experiences allow the formation of an early therapeutic relationship and the student is motivated to learn, it is likely that a successful outcome will result in spite of previous traumas and psychological reverses.

3. If, on the other hand, early life experiences have been so destructive that positive human relationships have not been able to take place and, as a result, strong neurotic and characterological defenses have been established (evident in the therapy by negativism, hostility, and strong resistance), it is likely that psychotherapy will result in failure or only modest gains. The therapist who responds to such students with a negative countertransference, as noted through coldness, withdrawal, and various forms of rejection, will serve only to reinforce a self-fulfilling prophesy on the part of the patient. A poor outcome often with premature termination is likely to occur.

4. While therapist characteristics are important, notably the ability to provide a nurturant environment, to control countertransference reactions, and expertise in facilitating therapeutic learning, these variables are not sufficient in themselves to overshadow student variables.

5. The experienced psychotherapists utilized in Strupp's studies were psychoanalytically trained and worked from this theoretical framework. Thus, those students who had successful outcomes were determined as being comfortable with the orientation offered by their therapists. They were also satisfied with the time limits of brief therapy and were able to work within this time frame. The author challenges the counseling and psychotherapeutic community to devise psychological interventions that are more practical for those students who are not amenable to traditional short-term counseling and psychotherapy.

Strupp's (1980a, 1980b, 1980c) research has been corroborated in large part by a recent investigation by Hill et al. (1983). The principal author conducted 12 sessions of individual insight-oriented counseling with a 20-year-old female student. Presenting problems included difficulties with her boyfriend and family, anxiety, and headaches. The therapeutic intervention involved interpretation, confrontation, the use of Gestalt techniques and discussion of the client-therapist relationship. A wider range of outcome and process measures was utilized. Sessions were of 60-minutes duration and all were conducted behind a one-way mirror and were audiotaped for purposes of analysis by judges. Results confirmed previous research that client motivation and the ability to

profit from the counseling relationship were important for
successful outcome. Following an initial establishment of
rapport, process measures indicated that client change
appeared to be the result of interpretations, direct feedback,
Gestalt activities and discussion of the therapeutic relationship. Outcome measures showed that treatment was generally
positive and resulted in improvement after the 12 sessions.
However, although this improvement was maintained following
two months, the client relapsed at the end of seven months.
The authors concluded that therapy was too brief for this
student. It was complicated by a high level of story-telling
behavior, the fact that insight began to take place only
during the final stages of therapy and that there were too
many issues to deal with in the time limit established.

What can be concluded from research about the effectiveness of brief counseling and psychotherapy with students?
Several considerations are offered:

1. Outcome studies, whether based on measures of client
satisfaction, therapist ratings, or a combination thereof,
present convincing evidence of the effectiveness of brief
treatment. While methodological considerations have been
questioned and the low percent of return rate on satisfaction
questionnaires is particularly bothersome in some investigations, the overall positive results cannot be ignored.

2. Individual case studies, while offering less sanguine
results than traditional outcome research, appear to present
a very promising source for future investigation. In-depth
analyses have the potential of highlighting the specific
strengths and weaknesses of brief treatment.

3. Individual case studies underscore observations that
have been culled from clinical experience. These can be
summarized as follows: (a) some patients benefit from brief
treatment, some do not. Students who are highly motivated,
who are psychologically minded and who have substantial ego
strength based on a relatively healthy previous history, and
who are able to take advantage of what the therapist has to
offer are likely to be successful in therapy; (b) students
with multiple psychological issues and/or those with strongly
ingrained neurotic and characterological defenses are unlikely
to benefit from brief treatment; (c) a negative transference
(obviously) impedes a productive psychotherapy outcome; and,
(d) traditional insight-oriented brief psychotherapy is not
beneficial to all students. Some require longer periods of
therapy in order to incorporate beneficial effects, or a different, perhaps more practical, intervention.

SUMMARY

This chapter has attempted to present an overview of the
current state of brief counseling and psychotherapy with
students. It is based on our experiences at Duke University's
Counseling and Psychological Services and includes case illustrations in combination with the clinical and empirical observations of others.

Brief counseling and psychotherapy has been in evidence
since the days university mental health services began.
During the 1950s and early 1960s references to brief and
short-term treatment began to appear in the literature. A
large number of surveys reflect on the brevity of the number
of sessions. It is asserted that brief treatment is compatible with college students, reasons including the need for
autonomy and control, motivation for and expectation of
treatment, the nature of the developmental crises, and general
satisfaction with a brief number of visits.

Student selection variables are addressed. Motivation, a
relatively healthy ego, psychological mindedness together with
a willingness to accept interpretation, and the ability to
establish a rapid and positive realtionship with the therapist
are considered essential characteristics for determining
suitability for brief work. Therapist selection characteristics include belief in the effectiveness of brief therapy,
comfort with the position of authority, satisfaction with
modest goals, and the ability to make a rapid and accurate
assessment while establishing an early and positive relationship with the student. Therapist functions involve assisting
the student in defining the nature of the problem, maintaining
a focus, encouraging ventilation, and promoting insight.

A recent consideration involving the use of very brief
intervention and psychotherapy is described and applications
are outlined. These include reviewing and approving psychological work already done and/or affirming a psychological
decision already made, clarifying a diagnostic concern, environmental stress management, and promoting insight.

Finally, the question of the effectiveness of brief
counseling and psychotherapy is addressed. Traditional outcome studies and individual case investigations are reviewed.
The former present consistent evidence of favorable results.
Individual case studies confirm current clinical observations
--namely, while some students benefit from brief counseling
and psychotherapy, some do not. Factors relating to favorable
outcomes include motivation, psychological mindedness, ego
strength, and the ability to work within the therapist's frame
of reference. While therapist variables are important (the
ability to establish a nurturant and benign relationship,
control negative transference, and employ techniques to enhance therapeutic learning), these characteristics are not, in
themselves, sufficient to override patient variables.

REFERENCES

Adelstein, D.M., C.J. Gelso, J.R. Haws, K.G. Reed, and S.B. Spiegel. "The Change Process Following Time-Limited Therapy." In *Explorations in Time-Limited Counseling and Psychotherapy*, edited by C.J. Gelso and D.H. Johnson. New York: Teachers College, Columbia University, 1983.

Alexander, F. and T.M. French. *Psychoanalytic Therapy*. New York: Ronald Press, 1946.

Allen, D.A. and J. Janowitz. "A Study of the Outcome of Psychotherapy in a University Mental Health Service." *Journal of the American College Health Association* 13 (1964):361-378.

Arnstein, R.L. "Psychotherapy Quality Assessment. Part Three: Discussion." *Journal of the American College Health Association* 28 (1979):131-139.

Binder, J.L. and S. Weiskopf. "Facilitating Ego Mastery in Brief Psychotherapy with Medical Students." *American Journal of Psychotherapy* 29 (1975):575-592.

Blaine, G.B. "Short-Term Psychotherapy with College Stuents." *New England Journal of Medicine* 256 (1957):208-211.

Bloom, B.L. "Focused Single-Session Therapy: Initial Development and Evaluation." In *Forms of Brief Therapy*, edited by S.H. Budman. New York: The Guilford Press, 1981.

Blos, P. "Psychological Counseling of College Students. *American Journal of Orthopsychiatry* 16 (1946):571-580.

Brown, B.M., M. Binder, and K. Johannessen. "Brief Psychiatric Treatment and Symptom Improvement in University Students." *Journal of the American College Health Association* 28 (1980):330-335.

Butcher, J.N. and M.P. Koss. "Research on Brief and Crisis-Oriented Therapies." In *Handbook of Psychotherapy and Behavior Change: An Empirical Analysis*, 2nd ed., edited by S.L. Garfield and A.E. Bergin. New York: John Wiley and Sons, 1978.

Caplan, G. *Principles of Preventive Psychiatry*. New York: Basic Books, 1964.

Carlson, H.B. "Characteristics of an Acute Confusional State in College Students." *American Journal of Psychiatry* 114 (1958):900-909.

Chassell, J. "Individual Counseling of College Students." *Journal of Consulting Psychology* 4 (1940):205-209.

Davanloo, H. "A Method of Short-Term Dynamic Psychotherapy." In *Short-Term Dynamic Psychotherapy*, edited by H. Davanloo. New York: Jason Aronson, 1980.

Dorosin, D., J. Gibbs, and L. Kaplan. "Very Brief Interventions--A Pilot Evaluation." *Journal of the American College Health Association* 24 (1976):191-194.

Dunn, R.F., J.R. Lanning, V.D. Patch, and J.B. Sturrock. "The College Mental Health Center: A Report after Ten Years." *Journal of the American College Health Association* 28 (1980):321-325.

Faries, M. "Short-Term Counseling at the College Level." *Journal of Counseling Psychology* 2 (1955):182-184.

Farnsworth, D.L. *Psychiatry, Education, and the Young Adult.* Springfield, Ill.: Charles C. Thomas, 1966.

Frank, J.D. "Therapeutic Components of Psychotherapy: A 25-Year Progress Report of Research." *The Journal of Nervous and Mental Disease* 159 (1974):325-342.

Friedman, W.H. and F.W. Coons. "The Mental Health Unit of a Student Health Service: A Study of a Clinic." *Journal of the American College Health Association* 17 (1969): 270-283.

Funkenstein, D.H., editor. *The Student and Mental Health: An International View.* Cambridge: The Riverside Press, 1959.

Garfield, S.L. "Research on Client Variables in Psychotherapy." In *Handbook of Psychotherapy and Behavior Change: An Empirical Analysis*, 2nd ed., edited by S.L. Garfield and A.E. Bergin. New York: John Wiley and Sons, 1978.

Garfield, S.L. and M. Wolpin. "Expectations Regarding Psychotherapy." *Journal of Nervous and Mental Disease* 137 (1963):353-362.

Gelso, C.J. and D.H. Johnson, editors. *Explorations in Time-Limited Counseling and Psychotherapy.* New York: Teachers College, Columbia University, 1983a.

Gelso, C.J. and D.H. Johnson. "A Summing Up: Toward an Understanding of the Process and Outcomes of Time-Limited Therapy." In *Explorations in Time-Limited Counseling and Psychotherapy*, edited by C.J. Gelso and D.H. Johnson. New York: Teachers College, Columbia University, 1983b.

Gelso, C.J., S.B. Spiegel, and D.H. Mills. "Clients' and Counselors' Reactions to Time-Limited and Time-Unlimited Counseling." In *Explorations in Time-Limited Counseling and Psychotherapy*, edited by C.J. Gelso and D.H. Johnson. New York: Teachers College, Columbia University, 1983.

Glasscote, R.M. and M.E. Fishman. *Mental Health on the Campus*. Washington, D.C.: Joint Information Service of the American Psychiatric Association, 1973.

Goodheart, C.D. "Training Clinicians for Brief Dynamic Psychotherapy." Paper read at the 90th Annual Meeting of the American Psychological Association (symposium entitled The Delivery of Dynamic Brief Psychotherapy in a College Setting), August 25, 1982, Washington, D.C.

Gundle, S. and A. Kraft. "Mental Health Programs in American Colleges and Universities." *Bulletin of the Menninger Clinic* 20 (1956):57-69.

Gurman, D.L. and T. Gordon. "The Counseling Center at the University of Chicago." *American Psychologist* 3 (1948): 166-171.

Haggerty, J.L., B.A. Baldwin, and M.B. Liptzin. "Very Brief Interventions in College Mental Health." *Journal of the American College Health Association* 28 (1980):326-29.

Hanfmann, E. *Effective Therapy for College Students*. Washington, D.C.: Jossey-Bass, 1978.

Hill, C.E., J.A. Carter, and M.K. O'Farrell. "A Case Study of the Process and Outcome of Time-Limited Counseling." *Journal of Counseling Psychology* 30 (1983):3-18.

Ichikawa, A. "Observations of College Students in Acute Distress." *Student Medicine* 10 (1961):184-191.

Jacobs, M.A., J.J. Muller, H.D. Eisman, J. Knitzer, and A. Spilken. "The Assessment of Change in Distress Level and Styles of Adaptation as a Function of Psychotherapy." *Journal of Nervous and Mental Disease* 145 (1968):405-419.

Keilson, M.V., F.H. Dworkin, and C.J. Gelso. "The Effectiveness of Time-Limited Psychotherapy in a University Coun-

seling Center." *Journal of Clinical Psychology* 35 (1979):
631-636.

Keithly, L.J., S.J. Samples, and H.H. Strupp. "Patient
Motivation as a Predictor of Process and Outcome in
Psychotherapy." *Psychotherapy and Psychosomatics* 33
(1980):87-97.

Lorian, R.P. "Patient and Therapist Variables in the Treatment of Low-Income Patients." *Psychological Bulletin* 81
(1974):344-354.

Love, R.L. and H. Widen. "Short-Term Dynamic Psychotherapy:
Another Kind of Learning on Campus." Paper read at the
60th Annual Meeting of the American College Health Association, Section on Mental Health, April 14-17, 1982,
Seattle, Washington.

Malan, D.H. *A Study of Brief Psychotherapy.* London: Tavis-
stock, 1963.

---. *The Frontier of Brief Psychotherapy.* New York: Plenum,
1976.

Mann, J. *Time Limited Psychotherapy.* Cambridge, Mass.:
Harvard University Press, 1973.

Mann, J. and R. Goldman. *A Casebook in Time-Limited Psychotherapy.* New York: McGraw-Hill, 1982.

Marmor, J. "Short-Term Dynamic Psychotherapy." *The American
Journal of Psychiatry* 136 (1979):149-155.

Menninger, K.A. and P.S. Holzman. *Theory of Psychoanalytic
Technique.* New York: Basic Books, 1973.

Nash, E.H., R. Hoehn-Saric, C.C. Battle, A.R. Stone, S.D.
Imber, and J.D. Frank. "Systematic Preparation of
Patients for Short-Term Psychotherapy. II: Relation to
Characteristics of Patient, Therapist and the Psychothera-
peutic Process." *The Journal of Nervous and Mental
Disease* 140 (1965):374-383.

National Center for Health Statistics. *Characteristics of
Patients of Selected Types of Medical Specialists and
Practitioners: United States July 1963-June 1964.* Pub-
lication no. 1000, series 10, no. 28. Washington, D.C.:
Public Health Service, 1966.

Nigl, A. and S. Weiss. "Effects of Presenting Symptom and
Therapist Orientation on Treatment Outcome: A Followup

Study of Brief Therapy with College Students." *Journal of the American College Health Association* 24 (1976):203-207.

Pinkerton, R.S. and W.J.K. Rockwell. "One or Two Session Psychotherapy with University Students." *Journal of the American College Health Association* 30 (1982):159-162.

Podolnick, E.E., H.L. Pass, and D.M. Bybee. "A Psychodynamic Approach to Brief Therapy." *Journal of the American College Health Association* 28 (1979):109-113.

Poey, K. "Quality Assessment Study of Brief Psychotherapy at a University HMO Setting." *Journal of the American College Health Association* 30 (1981):135-138.

Posin, H.I. "Approaches to Brief Psychotherapy in a University Health Service." *Seminars in Psychiatry* 1 (1969): 399-404.

Rockwell, W.J.K. and R.S. Pinkerton. "Single-Session Psychotherapy." *American Journal of Psychotherapy* 36 (1982): 32-40.

Sarnat, J.E. "Psychotherapy Quality Assessment. Part II: Psychotherapy Quality Assessment via Record Review." *Journal of the American College Health Association* 28 (1979):131-139.

Sifneos, P.E. "Psychoanalytically Oriented Short-Term Dynamic or Anxiety-Provoking Psychotherapy for Mild Obsessional Neuroses." *Psychiatric Quarterly* 60 (1966):271-282.

———. "'The Motivational Process': A Selection for Prognostic Criterion for Psychotherapy of Short Duration." *Psychiatric Quarterly* 42 (1968):271-280.

———. "Change in Patients' Motivation for Psychotherapy." *American Journal of Psychiatry* 128 (1971):74-77.

———. *Short-Term Psychotherapy and Emotional Crisis.* Cambridge, Mass.: Harvard University Press, 1972.

———. "Motivation for Change." In *Short-Term Dynamic Psychotherapy*, edited by H. Davanloo. New York: Jason Aronson, 1980.

Socarides, C.W. "On the Usefulness of Extremely Brief Psychoanalytic Contacts. *Psychoanalytic Review* 41 (1954): 340-346.

Speers, R.X. "Brief Psychotherapy with College Women: Technique and Criteria for Selection." *American Journal of Orthopsychiatry* 32 (1962):434-444.

Strupp, H.H. "Success and Failure In Time-Limited Psycho-Therapy: A Systematic Comparison of Two Cases: Comparison 1." *Archives of General Psychiatry* 37 (1980a):395-603.

---. "Success and Failure in Time-Limited Psychotherapy: A Systematic Comparison of Two Cases: Comparison 2." *Archives of General Psychiatry* 37 (1980b):708-716.

---. "Success and Failure in Time-Limited Psychotherapy: Further Evidence: Comparison 4." *Archives of General Psychiatry* 37 (1980c):947-954.

Strupp, H.H. and S.W. Hadley. "Specific versus Nonspecific Factors in Psychotherapy: A Controlled Study of Outcome." *Archives of General Psychiatry* 36 (1979):1125-1136.

Weber, D.J. and D.H. Tilley. "Patients' Evaluation of the Mental Health Service at a Health Sciences Campus." *Journal of the American College Health Association* 29 (1981):193-194.

Wedge, B.M., editor. *Psychosocial Problems of College Men.* New Haven: Yale University Press, 1958.

Whittington, H.G. "Transference in Brief Psychotherapy: Experience in a College Psychiatric Clinic." *Psychiatric Quarterly* 36 (1962):503-518.

Wolberg, L.R. *Short-Term Psychotherapy.* New York: Grune and Stratton, 1965.

---. *Handbook of Short-Term Psychotherapy.* New York: Thieme-Stratton, 1980.

2

Self Psychology and a Perspective on Psychological Issues

Joseph E. Talley

My working definition of *self psychology* is very broad
and is an amalgamation of a number of ideas woven together in
a manner that seems to fit well theoretically and to match
experiential observations in psychotherapy. The basic ideas
have come from many writing clinicians, particularly Fair-
bairn, Jung, Erik Erickson, Mahler, and Kohut. Such a weav-
ing together is not entirely unique or original, but I have
found this conceptual framework to be of considerable value
in treating late adolescents and young adults with emotional
difficulties. Undoubtedly some from particular schools of
thought will disagree with the selection of certain technical
terms as these terms are often used in a variety of ways. It
is my aim, for the sake of clarity, to be as simple as possible in choosing terms and expressions. Consequently, it
may appear at times that I presume a somewhat elementary
point needs more clarification than, in fact, it does. Although there is nothing esoteric to be offered, the components of this framework have not generated a great amount of
literature specifically in the area of psychotherapy with
students.

The purpose of this chapter is to present some related
concepts that will add a dimension (or further develop an
existing one) to the psychotherapist's approach with students.
This framework need not exclude the use of Gestalt, Cognitive-
Behavioral, Psychoanalytic, or other techniques, since the
aim is primarily to assist in the assessment of conditions
for which a variety of interventions or techniques may be
used. The focus will be on two levels: the content of the
self and the capacity of the self. Other specific developmental issues, such as the formation of a sexual identity,
described in the chapter on the treatment of grief, may be

viewed as particular aspects of the more general areas of development described in this chapter.

CONTENT OF THE SELF

The content of the self may be thought of as being comprised of multiple selves and as Horowitz and Zilberg (1983) write, "The 'I' of one state of mind is not necessarily the same as the 'I' of a person's next state of mind." There are varying degrees of cleavage between one self and the next and when a person's central locus of perception is in one self, the individual may have only a slight awareness (if any at all) of how it would feel to experience this moment through the eyes of a different internal self state. The different inner selves (or "voices") may be conceptualized as the internalized representations of significant others. These internalizations usually include feelings about the self, others, and the world, as well as schemata concerning how to act in relation to others. The thinking and perceiving self, often called the ego or "supraordinate self" (Horowitz and Zilberg 1983), may for any number of reasons identify, cathect, or become attached to a given internalization at any time. The experience of consciousness is comprised of these inner fluctuations. While attached to one self the ego may be quite blind to the thoughts and feelings of another self. Then for usually unknown reasons the ego becomes attached to or is overshadowed by another self, and feelings and thoughts change. This may all sound like multiple personality, and if the ego were totally engulfed by an internalization then such a form of profound dissociation would exist. However, it can be said that we each do have multiple personalities of sorts but that the degree of dissociation involved is most often very subtle and almost imperceptible. This phenomenon appears similar to what the Transactional Analysts call "ego states."

During our lives then, we are engaged in a process of internalizing others that are important to us and since humans are more impressionable when younger, the most potent internalizations are in all likelihood formed during childhood. The mother internalization, for example, includes not only vivid images of one's mother but also some associations concerning how the mother felt about the child and what might be called a set of "programs," "tapes," or "beliefs" about the world. The internalized mother representation also includes constellations of thought and feeling about the child in relation to the world (relationship paradigms) as well as a set of values concerning how things ought to be (the ego ideal).

To make matters more complex, this internalization has clusters around "bad" and "good." That is to say that there is a cluster of mother images that have painful or frustrating associations making up the "bad mother" image and a cluster of images around the pleasant and gratifying experiences constituting the "good mother" image. There is also a "good self" image *vis à vis* mother and a "bad self" image *vis à vis* mother. Further, a number of possible vicissitudes exist thematically within this internalization (for example, good mother, bad self seeing the world as bad but trying to correct it and in so doing correct the self; versus bad mother, good self seeing the world as bad but trying to correct it and in so doing correct mother). Given the number of elements in any internalization the thematic possibilities based on various combinations are formidable. It is apparent that the number of possible vicissitudes in relation to one internalization might keep life busy enough, but in multiplying the number of possible variations on the theme by the number of internalizations it is obvious why understanding the self at any level of depth is difficult. Likewise it should be apparent that forming a consistent sense of "I" really is an accomplishment. In order to achieve a unified sense of "I" the ego must have sufficient fortitude to regulate the internalizations currently vying for control. Of course in most persons this develops without any conscious intention. The ego in this instance is the sense of self that can become sufficiently detached from the magnetic-like pull of various internalizations to adequately reconcile the multiple internal selves so that the individual has the capacity for certain endeavors or developmental tasks.

CAPACITY OF THE SELF

These endeavors include the separation/individuation of the self, the further consolidation of the self, the regulation of self-esteem, and the union of the self with another, or intimacy. I refer to these tasks as endeavors here because it lends a more affective quality. To call them "phases" or "stages" implies a more exclusively sequential process than appears necessarily to be the case. However, the work does seem to have for the most part a sequential nature to it, although activity is probably occurring in more than one area at a time and there may be a periodic "turning back" to work again in a certain area. Further, some differences in "levels" may exist. For example, in order to achieve a sense of separation from parents, some sense of self must already exist but a much finer clarification of the self can occur after a sense of separation has been achieved. Clearly the first differentiation is at a deeper level than the later clarification. Other complications include the integration of Heinz Kohut's (]977) "bipolar self" and self-esteem with the other tasks since questions exist regarding at what "level" these distinctions occur. Nevertheless, it is clear that students often present with disturbances in the area of self-esteem including motivational (ambition) problems and concomitant dilemmas about values (ideals). These are the basic self issues.

Although this framework may seem unduly cumbersome for brief therapy, an in-depth accurate assessment is necessary for any therapeutic strategy that goes beyond trial and error. There is no pretense that all of the endeavors or tasks can be addressed in brief therapy or that a "mini-analysis" can be done. Nevertheless, I would suggest that if an adequate assessment is made, various interventions might be brought to bear at the point of the student's present impasse and once over that impasse, the natural push toward growth and development will keep the momentum going for varying periods of time. This presumes that the student does not have a thought disorder, a borderline personality, manic-depressive illness, and does not for some other reason absolutely require long-term treatment. Yet, even those for whom longer term treatment does seem the ideal option, well done brief therapy can generally be of significant benefit.

Separating the Self

The late adolescent and young adult are usually experiencing increased psychological if not geographic distance from parents. As the responsibilities of adult life become clearer, the student may have very mixed feelings regarding the loss of a position that allows some degree of dependence on the parents. Since what is acted out often resembles the darting away from and sudden running back to the mother, described by Mahler, Pine, and Bergman (1975) as common to children between 18 and 36 months going through the separation/individuation from mother phase, we might view the student as in the process of reworking these feelings once again. (Presumably a reworking would have occurred around puberty also.) However, during the earlier work on separation/individuation the resulting awareness was of being "separate and dependent," but, the reworking during young adulthood should result in the awareness of being "separate and independent." Mahler, Pine, and Bergman's (1975) description of the child's experience does not sound too unlike that of late adolescence and young adulthood: "There are periods in which the child feels exuberently omnipotent, interspersed with states of extreme sobriety or depression during which the child feels helpless and longs for the lost world."

Austin and Inderbitzin (1983) have emphasized this point and offer case reports on the "recapitulation" of separation/individuation issues in their student mental health experience and how this issue can serve as the focus of treatment.

During such episodes the wish for autonomy coupled with the fear of abandonment are salient.

Case Example. A was a 21-year-old male engineering student from the Midwest and was beginning his junior year after a leave of absence. He came seeking help for increasing anxiety about his academic work as he had done the preceding year after a few weeks of classes. At that time he wished to be away from school for a year, thinking that taking this time off and working would allow him to return with more confidence. A had taken some courses at a college in his hometown during the year also and he had experienced no problematic anxiety. He described the support he received from his mother as keeping him "pumped up" enough to do the work, as was the case in high school. Further history taking of the motivational problem revealed that A had had a girlfriend two years his senior for his first two years of college. She admittedly kept him "pumped up" also and was supportive like his mother, whom the girl reportedly resembled. Returning to school, after the girlfriend had graduated, left A feeling very alone and helpless. Both women had pushed him toward an engineering career.

In two sessions A was talking about his dependency on his mother as well as the desire to please her and soon he saw that this scenario was replayed with his girlfriend. By the eighth session he was talking about leaving engineering for subjects he truly felt interest in, and by the twelfth session he had done this and no longer wished to be "dependent on a psychologist" since the anxiety was not currently a problem.

Although several issues are prominent in this case, the differentiation of the self from parents and their representations was fundamental. Anxiety subsided as A asserted his independence.

Increased Consolidation of the Self

Erik Erickson (1968) writes:

Various selves . . . make up our composite self. There are constant and often shock-like transitions between these selves: consider the nude body self in the dark suddenly exposed in the light; consider the clothed self among friends or in the company of higher-ups or lower downs; consider the just awakened drowsy self or the one stepping refreshed out of the surf or the one overcome by retching and fainting; the body self in sexual excitement or rage; the competent self and the impotent one; the one on horseback, the

> *one in the dentist's chair. . . . It takes,*
> *indeed, a healthy person for the "I" to speak*
> *out of all of these conditions in such a way*
> *that at any given moment it can testify to a*
> *reasonably coherent Self.*

Erickson's description relates more to social roles and certain variations in feeling common to all persons whereas a deeper sense of self fragmentation is seen in Kohut's statement, "We recognize the simultaneous existence of contradictory selves: of different selves of various degrees of stability and of various degrees of importance" (Kohut 1977).

In their paper, "On the Adolescent Process as a Transformation of the Self," Wolf, Gedo, and Terman (1977) conclude that the nuclear self (the one most resistant to change) is tested in its self-assertive and idealistic dimensions during adolescence, and under "favorable circumstances" a "significant firming" occurs. The increased consolidation of the self (done consciously or unconsciously) remains a necessary endeavor of young adulthood since without it sustained, comfortable intimacy is impossible because close relationships will become little more than the acting out of projections arising from unmastered internalizations.

In consolidating the self, greater mastery is achieved if the selves relating to both "masculine" and "feminine" aspects as well as selves representing certain Jungian archetypes are integrated in the personality. Such theoretical abstractions can be made very relevant to the young adult with questions like, "If you would imagine yourself as being of the opposite sex, what would you be like? . . . How would that make things different now? . . . What scenario comes to mind if you think of yourself as a hero(ine)? . . . Can you describe the aspect of your self most related to shame and revulsion? . . . Can you imagine yourself as a wise old man? . . . A healing, soothing mother?" Through the activation of the various symbolic selves, movement towards the consolidation of the self is enhanced. The academically-oriented young adult usually responds well to this type of self-development and may also become more conscious of the process, whereas the less academically-minded person might achieve this development while painting, playing music, or building a house and never need to process the experience verbally at all. The student's bringing in dreams for a few sessions can aid immensely in this type of effort toward consolidation and integration.

Often the activation of a symbolic self that has been cut off from the rest of conscious experience can establish a more harmonious equilibrium. For example, developing a clear image of an assertive or appropriately aggressive self with its associated emotions, such as the warrior in battle, may permit assertive behavior that had been heretofore inhibited.

Case Example. R was a 19-year-old male undergraduate who had recently shown a marked decrement in academic performance. As he talked he repeatedly complained about how "competitive" his peers were and said that he did not wish to be "so aggressive." He had done very well in high school and college until the time came to declare a major. R clearly viewed this as joining the adult world because it would influence his career options.

Further assessment revealed that he had recently begun to "feel guilty about being competitive" in intramural basketball, and because of this was not playing as well as he once had. Although R had never been particularly aggressive in athletics or academics, he was now being quite passive and felt that it would somehow be wrong to act otherwise. He was the youngest of three sons born to a "cold and intimidatingly aggressive" father who was an attorney and a "self-sacrificing and somewhat passive" mother. The oldest brother, also an attorney, had, along with the father, verbally abused the mother frequently. The second brother, who had also attended law school but was a business entrepreneur, was seen as "a man of action" and more distant from the family, while R was closest to his mother and admittedly identified with her, adopting her view that "aggressiveness is bad."

During the first three sessions R concluded that he had wished to avoid being like his father because of the father's criticism of both R and his mother. Subsequent work with early memories and imagery allowed R to recall times when the father had shown a supportive interest in him and times when the mother had induced some family problems. With a more balanced set of memories R was able to consider that his father might have some worthwhile qualities and that even aggressiveness, if channeled into appropriate self-assertion and competitiveness, might have some merit. After a few more sessions R began to comment on the therapist's periodic directiveness while nevertheless showing personal concern and a supportive interest. Soon R concluded that being competitive or assertive need not also include being cold or critical toward others.

With his healthy assertiveness now accessible to the rest of the personality, R's performance in several spheres improved. Apparently the heightened passivity was brought on when he felt the pressure to choose a major. To him this was equated with the push to join the adult (competitive) world, thus requiring him to be more aggressive which did not agree with his values at that time. Moreover, the choosing of a major highlighted the fact that all of the men in his family had attended law school and now he must reckon with whether to choose a major compatible with law school or break with the tradition of the men in his family. R's initial reaction was

to deny the aspects of himself that he saw as similar to
the father and brothers. Increased consolidation of the
self enabled R to cope with the ambivalence resulting from
the opposing pulls of the mother and father internalizations.

Self-Esteem

Students presenting for help with deflated (and sometimes
inflated) self-esteem are a regular occurrence at our service. Initially it must be ascertained whether the disturbance is reactive to a recent event or if poor self-esteem is
a state of long duration. Heinz Kohut (1977) sees self-
esteem as a function of what he terms "the bipolar self."
This bipolarity places ambition at one end and values or
ideals at the other. The solidifying of these poles results
in a person ambitiously and creatively pursuing work that is
guided by ideals. Kohut's psychoanalytic method informed by
Self Psychology is, as he presents it, for use in long-term
treatment particularly for persons with narcissistic disorders. For a profound disturbance in self-esteem that has
for many years thwarted productivity and enjoyment in work or
personal relationships, long-term therapy does appear to be the
treatment of choice. However, it seems that Kohut's bipolar
self does have relevance to brief therapy also.
Some work toward the consolidation of ideals and ambitions can be done in brief psychotherapy. In fact, vocational counseling serves this end and in dealing with psychosocial problems, the development of appropriate assertiveness
may do the same. No claim is made that a new self "structure"
will result from brief therapy but experience as well as
theory suggest that increased consolidation of the existing
self is possible in brief treatment (see Chapter 1). The
very factors that normally, according to Kohut, are operative
in development and result in positive self-esteem are also
elements of good brief therapy. Two primary developmental
factors are involved. First, exhibitionism is transformed
into ambition by the mother's empathy with or the "mirroring"
of exhibitionistic and grandiose manifestations followed by
her responsiveness gradually becoming more appropriate to
reality. Second, the child's value system is begun by the
parents' toleration of the child's idealization of them followed by a gradual period of de-idealization.
In brief treatment, hopefully, the therapist is highly
empathic and will show initial acceptance of any mild to
moderate exhibitionistic or grandiose thinking that is not
indicative of a thought disorder. Such "acceptance" may be
followed by a tolerable and appropriate decrease of displayed
empathy with extremes so that the therapist's response comes
to match more closely what others in the world might offer.

Further, the student very well may initially idealize the therapist and if the therapist will accept (not to imply encourage) the idealization, then a healthy identification of sorts may still remain after the de-idealization process. Thus, the bulk of Kohut's conditions for the development of self-esteem can be recreated at least in part in brief psychotherapy. The transference, of course, can only be addressed minimally in brief work.

In short, if the therapist is attuned to self disturbances it is likely that some progress can be made in brief therapy. This would be most noticeable when a skill that can build and generalize, such as being more assertive, is developed. A note of caution: Significant disturbances in self-esteem often are erroneously treated as developmental anxieties common to the "college years." This results in the student later feeling a lack of readiness to leave the protection found in being a student.

Case Example. H was a 19-year-old sophomore who presented as very soft-spoken and shy. Her affect was flat and she indicated that her mother had been hospitalized for depression several times. H felt so inhibited in groups that she would not speak out and this resulted in lowered self-esteem, since she felt she contributed nothing and that her friends must find her boring. On the other hand, she would at times feel superior and act aloof.

It emerged in a few sessions that as a little girl, H would try to keep her mother from becoming depressed by amusing her. When this failed and the mother became worse, H felt that her mother was indicating that H was not enough to keep her happy. H never was able to share this frustration with her mother. This fit very well with the picture of the mother as a highly critical, meticulous woman. H's posture psychologically was "good" mother, "bad" self accepting that "my efforts to help will be useless." However, a less frequently observed inner position also occurred that went something like, "Well, my conversation may not be very good but at least I know it and am good enough to feel bad about it, while you, my friends, often have very foolish things to say but you are too stupid to even feel bad about it." A certain smugness existed at these times when H identified with her mother and looked critically toward others as H assumed her mother had looked at her. A sense of self-righteousness about her guilt and self-criticism filled her showing the truth of the saying that "Guilt (often) kisses as it bites." The bite, of course, is the sense of inadequacy while the kiss is recognizing the "goodness" of feeling deservedly inadequate. Thus a small portion of self-esteem is preserved by identification with the internalized critic.

In a few sessions H became acutely aware of the inner voices she was yielding to, what the internalization included,

and the fact that she projected critical aspects of the
internalization onto friends while at other times she identified with it so much that she would view others quite
harshly. With the therapist's help, H accepted the idea
that in order to feel better she would have to diminish her
present method of feeling good (that is, self righteous
criticism of others and self righteousness about feeling so
critical of herself). Considering this shift in thinking
was initially difficult, but after 20 sessions she was
becoming much less critical of herself as well as others
and being much more outgoing in groups. She found this to
be fun and rewarding. When H felt less victimized by her
mother and able to be appropriately assertive with her
mother she was also able to feel more compassion for the
mother.

Intimacy and the Self

     The concern of, "What happens when we get close?" is
omnipresent on campuses. Uniting of the self with another,
establishing intimacy, requires a sense of trust in the
potency of self to come together with the other and not be
overpowered or engulfed by the other. Thus the belief that
separation can be regained and sufficient autonomy maintained is essential. Clearly, separation/individuation as
well as the consolidation of the self must be substantial
before intimacy or sustained union can be enjoyed. Consequently, attempted union prior to considerable mastery of
the other endeavors discussed is likely to result in a disturbed family (if marriage occurs) rather than a disturbed
person. Difficulty in this area is usually a sign to begin
work in the other areas, as a sense of trust in the basic
competence of the self as autonomous has, in all likelihood,
not been established.
     Obviously, it cannot be expected that a good intimate
relationship is possible between just any two randomly
selected people, and late adolescence and young adulthood
are times of clarifying what one wants in a partner and what
is actually possible to have. When perfectionistic "great
expectations" refuse to abate with age or when each romantic
relationship results in one party regressing to the point of
acting out a very childlike role, then intimacy is thwarted
in favor of replaying old issues. Moreover, what appears
to be an intimate relationship on the surface is often
fraught with unending criticism causing an emotional distance that demonstrates a lack of true acceptance and hence
a lack of real intimacy.
     If intimacy is actually desired, and frequently it is
not, then an eventual reckoning must come regarding the ques-

tion, "Are all the people I've dated really inadequate or am
I expecting too much?" If this is the problem area, then
psychotherapy may allow the student more control in choosing
between intimacy and a necessary decrease in the intensity
of critical internalizations or isolation and continued
identification with the internalized other as an empty substitute for intimacy.

A variation on this theme exists when the student proj-
ects the critical internalization onto others. Then it is
feared that if all is not well the partner will brutally
chastise and/or abandon the individual. Consequently, such
a fearful person may surrender all sense of will and independence in the relationship and wish only to comply with and
please the parentified lover. When it is recognized that
submissiveness is the result of getting close to another,
then closeness is feared and avoided.

Case Example. K, a 25-year-old female graduate student
in Economics from a Japanese-American family, found that
whenever she was emotionally close to a man she became almost
childlike in her efforts to please. Further, she could find
no fault with the man but continually worried about what
faults he might find in her. K's father was a "self-made
authoritarian type" and had been the only parent she could
rely on at all for physical or emotional nurturing. Her
mother was "always bedridden with one thing or another and
seemed to need more than she could give." In part due to the
mother's stance, the father's role became much more significant and his devoted personal attention felt like magic when
it was given. However, the father would also shift without
apparent warning and be harshly punitive and at times physi-
cally abusive. It was clear that the father was attempting
to create an emotional closeness with K to compensate for the
lack of intimacy he had with his wife. From this childhood
experience K learned, in effect, that intimacy with a man
results in domination. Her first solution to this was to
seek passive-dependent men for boyfriends who posed no threat
to father as the most powerful and significant man in her
life. Nevertheless, she did not respect these passive men
and therefore no real intimacy was established since she
played the parentified lover role with them. After an extended evaluation it appeared that K would benefit most from
long-term work in which the transference might be used extensively. Since this was financially possible for her, a referral was made.

In this case there was no marked ego strength deficit but
rather the emotionally impoverished childhood with the absence of a consistent nurturer that made long-term work the
treatment of choice. However, this is not to say that something worthwhile but more limited might not have been possible to accomplish in three to six months.

Conclusion

It should be evident that all of the developmental tasks or endeavors discussed are interrelated. Brief psychotherapy may work toward the increased differentiation of the student from the family of origin so that more independent feeling and thinking is possible. This accomplishment hopefully results in a more independent choice of vocation and mate. Thus the repetition of scenarios from the family of origin are minimized. The movement from a stage of separation/individuation to a stage of consolidation of the self (through the taming and integration of internalizations) seems to form a comfortable continuum resulting in the possibility of intimacy. However, Kohut's factor of self-esteem with the developmental components of solidified ideals and ambitions does not fit together as easily in a linear model since the development of self-esteem should occur simultaneously with the other tasks, but at a different level.

While more therapeutic work can usually be done in more time with self issues, and a certain number of more severely disturbed students do require long-term psychotherapy, the concepts presented here are also relevant for brief psychotherapy with less disturbed students. In such an approach the accurate assessment of the problematic developmental or self issue is fundamental. Students with adequate ego strength may benefit significantly from brief psychotherapy with such an accurate focus. Thus, understanding clinical observations from long-term psychotherapy and psychoanalysis regarding disturbances of self-esteem and the development of the self is beneficial for the brief treatment of students with whom global alteration of the personality is not necessary. This would primarily include students whose disturbances are not lifelong but who are currently suffering from a "bruised" sense of self-esteem or a developmental setback that is reactive to some event.

REFERENCES

Austin, L. and L. Inderbitzin. "Brief Psychotherapy in Late Adolescence: A Psychodynamic and Developmental Approach." *American Journal of Psychotherapy* 37 (1983):202-209.

Erikson, E. *Identity, Youth and Crisis*. New York: W. W. Norton, 1968.

Horowitz, M. and N. Zilberg. "Regressive Alterations of the Self Concept." *American Journal of Psychiatry* 140 (1983): 284-289.

Kohut, H. *The Restoration of the Self*. New York: International Universities Press, 1977.

Mahler, M., F. Pine, and A. Bergman. *The Psychological Birth of the Human Infant*. New York: Basic Books, 1975.

Wolf, E., J. Gedo, and D. Terman. "On the Adolescent Process as a Transformation of the Self." *Journal of Youth and Adolescence* 1:257-272.

3

Using Early Memories
in Brief Psychotherapy

Joseph E. Talley

This chapter will focus on two uses of early memories as
a tool for effecting change in university students. A preliminary empirical investigation with the use of one variation
of the technique will be presented along with hypotheses
generated by the data regarding what types of students might
respond best to the tool. A detailed description of the second variation will also be presented.

A brief review of the most relevant literature on early
memories will set the stage for the presentation of the study
and subsequent discussion.

EARLY WRITINGS

The first modern investigation of the meaning of early
memories was done by Sigmund Freud which culminated in his
1899 paper on "Screen Memories." Freud used the term "screen"
memories for these earliest memories because he found them to
function as screens that inhibited the recall of more dis-
turbing contiguous events. This conclusion was based on a
number of observations, among them that hysterics habitually
showed amnesia for some or all of the events leading to the
onset of symptoms, early memories were often found to be fic-
titious, forgotten elements of the memories became manifest
during psychoanalytic treatment, and memories were altered
over time as was evidenced by the fact that the subject in the
memory image often appeared as an object being observed.
Freud writes:

> It may indeed be questioned whether we have
> any memories at all from our childhood:
> memories relating to our childhood may be all

*that we possess. Our childhood memories
show us our earliest memories not as they
were but as they appear at later periods
when the memories were aroused. In these
periods of arousal, the child's memories
did not, as people are accustomed to say,
emerge; they were formed at that time.
And a number of motives, with no concern
for historical accuracy, had a part in
forming them, as well as in the selection
of the memories themselves [Freud 1899].*

Thus for Freud the early memory was significant because of
what it concealed more than for what it revealed. Yet it did
reveal something, according to Freud, as he believed the
memory to be closely associated with that material which was
suppressed, since it was selected to be remembered instead of
the suppressed material. Thus, the memory represents a compromise between what in fact did happen and the desire to
deny totally the traumatic event. It is also a symbolic
representation of the compromise made between the person's
impulses and taboos or between wishes and reality. Hence, a
primary therapeutic task for Freud was to uncover the "forgotten" elements behind the screen memory so that the origins
of the symptom might be understood, thus allowing the primary
conflict to be exposed and analyzed. In this framework the
screen memory is a defense as well as a compromise because it
protects against the unmasking of the primary conflict.

Alfred Adler, breaking from Freud, concluded that the
manifest content of the early memory was itself the key to
understanding one's life-style and particular inferiority
complex. He writes:

*When rightly understood in relation to the
rest of an individual's life, his early recollections are found always to have a bearing on
the central interests of that person's life.
Early recollections give us hints and clues
which are most valuable to follow when attempting the task of finding the directions of a
person's strivings. They are most helpful in
revealing what one regards as values to be
aimed for and what one senses as dangers to be
avoided. They help us to see the kind of world
which a particular person feels he is living
in and the ways he early found of meeting that
world [Adler 1937].*

Adlerians have continued to use early memories in this way.

DIAGNOSTIC USES

Since the laying of this early theoretical groundwork by Freud and Adler, others have followed with case reports describing how a particular patient's early memories related to his present life situation, and correlational studies have been done attempting to differentiate the content of early memories by patient diagnosis. For example, Eisenstein and Ryerson (1951) found that schizophrenic and borderline subjects had more autoerotic and sexual content in their early memories than did subjects diagnosed neurotic. The former were also more likely to be alone in the memory.
Stella Chess reports:

> The formation of the memory is firstly
> related to the needs of the child's memory
> at the time that the incident occurs, and
> secondly that the nature of the memory as
> it is recalled at some subsequent time, is
> dependent upon the needs of the personality
> at the time of recall [Chess 1951].

Thus, while focusing on the manifest content for diagnostic purposes, Chess continues with Freud's proposition that the memory is reconstructed to serve present needs. For these reasons the particular early memory recalled at a time of stress may reveal what the person's needs were in relation to that stressful event. Further, Chess emphasizes that the type and quality of interpersonal relationships in the memory divulge how the subject has chosen to see himself in relation to others. In his paper "The Diagnostic Importance of Early Recollections," agreeing with Chess, Paul Brodsky (1952) writes:

> The psychic function of this memory is to
> serve as a guide for approaching the problems
> of life. . . . In observing how the patient
> undertakes to produce these highly indicative
> early recollections, the therapist will find
> it useful to keep in mind the following diag-
> nostic criteria:
> (1) The patient's approach to the task of
> reproducing recollections. (Does the
> subject appear indifferent, self-assured,
> give only what is asked for, etc.?)
> (2) Indications of organ inferiorities and
> emotional tendencies.
> (3) The role the patient assigns to himself
> in the recollection.
> (4) The locale of the recollection.

(5) The role assigned to family members.
(6) The role assigned to others.

This information should leave the therapist with an impression of how the individual sees himself, the environment, and others.

Saul, Snyder, and Sheppard (1956) maintain a similar perspective and allege that early memories

> *. . . reveal, probably more clearly than any
> other single psychological datum, the central
> core of each person's psychodynamics, form of
> neurosis and emotional problem, . . . the*
> conditionability *of the human is so great and
> so sensitive during the very first months and
> years of life that emotional influences during
> them, particularly prolonged influences, are
> especially potent in shaping the personality
> for all the rest of life. The earliest memo-
> ries are probably the most powerful single
> device for penetrating to the essentials of
> the aftereffects of these influences.*

Lieberman (1957) investigated the use of early memories as a projective technique and found that memories including sex and punishment were more prevalent in psychotics than nonpsychotics. In an investigation with 400 psychiatric patients, it was found that schizophrenics recalled more memories in which they were the only person and in which the settings were unclear than did hysterics, while hysterics reported more themes of aggression, illness, rejection, moral issues, and travel (Langs, Rothenberg, Fishman, & Reiser 1960).

Mayman and Faris' (1970) paper "Early Memories as Expressions of Relationship Paradigms" offers illustrative case examples such as the following:

> *(Earliest memory?) My mother turned the hot
> water on instead of cold water in the sink.
> (?) She used to bathe me in the sink and she
> got the wrong water faucet, the hot water
> instead of the cold. (Other details?) I seem
> to remember telling her she turned the wrong
> faucet on, but I don't know whether I was able
> to talk or not. They said I had a large vocab-
> ulary at that time. I don't know . . . it
> seemed I was trying to get her not to turn
> that faucet on. (?) Just an honest mistake.
> It burned of course. (Age at the time?) That
> I don't know. I imagine between one and two.*

Inferences

Even as an inarticulate infant, he sees him-
self as taking over for the mother the care
of himself. He pictures himself as someone
who even in infancy was not a defenseless,
anaclitic, trusting child, but rather as some-
one who needed to look after himself. The
mother is represented tacitly as a thoughtless
woman who fails to care for him adequately.
The latent feeling is one of reproach against
the mother for her failure, and at the same
time a reaction formation against that re-
proach: It was, "just an honest mistake."

Burnell and Solomon (1964) attempted to predict success
or failure in basic military training on the basis of the
content of early memories. They discovered that trainees who
later became psychiatric patients reported a significantly
greater amount of aggressive action in their early memories.
The authors suggest that similar studies need to be done with
different populations such as college students. Although a
study conducted by Eva Dreikurs Ferguson (1964) revealed that
five judges were unable to achieve better than chance accuracy by using early memories to predict diagnosis, interjudge
reliability regarding diagnosis is in general problematic.
However, in the same study, interjudge reliability for life-
style predictions based on early memories was high.

Langs (1965) investigated the relationship between early
memory content and personality traits using projective tests
and social history as criteria. He found a significant relationship between the two with regard to aggression or hostility. Further, the subject's role in the memory was found to
be indicative of his present mode of coping.

Joshua Levy (1965) has attempted to organize a set of
units for scoring early memories utilizing such dimensions as
"active-passive, positive-negative, givingness, mastery and
neutrality," although to date no evidence regarding the
validity of combining these dimensions exists. In his article
"Early Memories and Character Structure," Martin Mayman (1968)
has continued in a similar mode by proposing several aspects
of the early memory's manifest content that need to be
assessed. These aspects include the following:

(1) relationship paradigms or the interper-
sonal context in which the subject describes
himself and the quality, intensity, and
psychosexual level of feelings toward others,
(2) coping style (is the subject passive or
active?),

(3) *self-structure or modalities (e.g.,*
sensual vs. *introspective) in which the*
person's feelings and experience are
most fully invested,

(4) *images and representations of significant*
others,

(5) *defense modes (e.g., repression, projec-*
tion, reaction-formation, etc.) and phobic,
depressive, self-punitive, withdrawn,
self-preoccupied themes vs. *warm and human*
cognitive-affective-behavioral constella-
tions.

Mayman allows for the analysis of both the manifest as well
as the latent content of the early memory and in so doing
permits the utility of not only the Freudian but also the
Adlerian model. However, this is done from an ego-psychology
vantage point that acknowledges the importance of unconscious
psychosexual content ignored by Adler. Mayman is also concerned with the defensive functions and object-relations
revealed, in part, in the manifest content. Finally, Mayman
proposes that when one cannot retrieve early experiences, the
patient's fantasies about "what might have happened" are not
only often as useful as a true recollection, but also frequently approximate what in reality did happen. Some case
studies of the use of this technique are described by Mayman
(1968) and also by Greve (1976).

Some differences between the sexes regarding early memories have been described. In one study (Adcock 1975), males
reported significantly more memories relating to games,
parties, accidents to self, and pleasurable experiences,
while females reported more memories relating to family interaction, frightening experiences, and sensual experiences.
This seems to be a questionable finding as some of the category descriptors are so similar (for example, pleasurable vs.
sensual).

TREATMENT USES

Shepard Gellert (1975) has reported psychotherapy case
studies in which the client was asked to "Play out the memory
as if it were now." Gellert's intent is to help the client
become aware of how present living is being influenced by
"decisions" that were made at an early age and subsequently
pushed out of awareness. This technique, born in Transactional Analysis, and currently known as "Redecision Therapy"
(Goulding & Goulding 1979), encourages the acting out of a
memory in which a decision was "made" or something learned
that has proven either to be not true or to have deleterious

effects on the person. The goal is to inculcate a new decision through reworking the memory. Finally, Binder and
Smokler (1980) have advocated the use of early memories as
a technique for the therapist to assess the type of conflict
and to select a focus for brief psychotherapy. They suggest
that the relating of the present conflict to an early memory
"illuminates the long standing importance of these feelings,
which serves to heighten motivation for treatment." Once
treatment is well underway the therapist will again refer to
the early memories in order to strengthen interpretations by
linking present maladaptive behavior to past experiences.
The sharing of early memories has been likened by Binder and
Smokler to "sharing the family photo album," thus building
rapport.

APPLICATION

It can be seen from the literature review that both diagnostic and treatment purposes can be served by the eliciting
of early memories. However, there are at least two variations to the approach. The first approach of straightfor-
wardly requestion the client's three or four earliest memories is perhaps best for diagnostic purposes and for treating
the more global personality issues of primary defense mechanisms and core conflicts. Therefore this strategy is most
likely best employed in moderate- to long-term therapy. This
method is applicable to briefer treatment for a specific presenting problem only in so far as the specific problem can be
related to the general personality issues in the client's
understanding.

Another variation of the use of early memories is to
elicit specific early memories associated with the presenting
troublesome feelings. The rationale for this technique lies
in the observation that painful events usually seem more
upsetting if they are similar to previous painful events.
For example, if a newly married student whose mother died
when he was a child is unfortunate enough to have his wife
die in an accident, the second loss may stir up feelings
about the first loss and thus the response to the second loss
may actually be a response to the combined effects of both
events. This will be particularly true if the former event
was and has remained emotionally walled off from the rest of
the man's conscious emotional experience. In this case the
latter event actually may prompt emotions more associated
with the first event. Thus, when the emotional response to
a current situation appears unusually exaggerated, it is very
likely that those emotions are at least in part the product
of an earlier experience. This process may be summarized as
"the rubber band effect" such that an elastic band held

stretched with one end in each hand may represent the link (that is, sadness about loss) between two events. When the second event actually occurs, the memory of the event at the other end of the link is shaken, thus releasing the associated feelings like a stretched rubber band that is released with one hand and stings the other. Likewise, present pain may be multiplied by an experience somehow being a repetition of an earlier frustrating event. The person may or may not be consciously aware of the event. Remembering the early event and experiencing the normal pain associated with it can therefore lessen its influences on current events. This method is more similar to Gellert's (1976) use.

The procedure may be initiated while listening to the details of the presenting complaint. As the associated affect escalates (assuming very good rapport), or at any time that affect associated with a current painful dilemma has built to what appears to be its peak, the therapist then interjects by asking gently but directly, "How do you feel right now?" (Pause for response.) "Can you tell me how you feel in specific parts of your body, your head, stomach, throat and shoulders?" (Pause for response.) Then the therapist says slowly and with a measured emphasis, "Now can you tell me the first time that you can remember feeling this way? Just picture the scene in your 'mind's eye' with as much detail and vividness as possible while you stay with the feeling. You may wish to close your eyes, but just take whatever comes up." This technique utilizes the momentum and access to the unconscious provided by the intense affect brought alive for the moment in a "safe" situation. This procedure should be repeated three or four times for the same focused concern in order to see the threads of similarity running through most of the memories. The entire process may be repeated for several focal conflicts over the course of treatment and may be combined with eliciting several of the earliest memories at the outset of therapy for diagnostic purposes as well as to relate them to memories about specific problems. In short, there is no reason for the methods to be mutually exclusive, although one may be better than the other for certain purposes.

A PRELIMINARY INVESTIGATION WITH STUDENTS

The findings reported in this investigation result from employing the first method that would in all probability be more difficult for the client to see as valuable in one session unless the presenting conflict could be easily related to the more general core conflicts. Thus, an investigation employing the second early memories procedure described would be a valuable supplement to the findings presented here. The results of this investigation suggest types of clients that might respond best to the first procedure. Summaries of the earliest memories for each subject are given as well as comments regarding the subsequent usage of the memories in brief treatment.

The preliminary investigation described below was designed to gather information about student reaction to the eliciting of earliest memories during the initial session and to determine with whom the technique was most effective. The criterion for efficacy was student evaluation. An evaluation questionnaire was employed to gather data regarding particulars associated with eliciting early memories in the initial session. Eliciting memories in the first session was consistent with Binder and Smokler's (1980) hypothesis that it would build rapport and enhance motivation by helping the student see that there may be connections between present dilemmas and earlier experiences. Thus the need for treatment would be made more evident as would the belief that the therapist could be of help.

METHOD

The subjects were 24 students between the ages of 18 and 28 who presented for counseling of a psychosocial nature at the University of Virginia's Counseling Center. There were 14 females and 10 males. Half the students of each sex were placed in the control group and half in the experimental group. The therapists were six doctoral students all doing their predoctoral internship at the agency. Four were men, two were women, and all had had similar amounts of prior experience and training. All therapists received brief training in the use of early memories and role-played the eliciting of early memories and sequence of questions designed to help the student connect the early memories to the present problem (see Appendix A).

Every therapist had two students in the control group (no memories requested) and two students in the experimental group (two earliest memories requested, "whichever one strikes you," at approximately 20 minutes into the session). The memories were intentionally requested after the student had been given some time to describe the current problem and establish a sense of comfort with the therapist.

A brief client satisfaction index (see Appendix B) was given to each student at the end of the session to be completed and placed anonymously in a box by the door as the student left. Age and sex were requested on the form. The control group received a form with questions one through six while the experimental group received a form with questions one through ten.

RESULTS AND DISCUSSION

The results are somewhat complicated by the fact that one person in the control group (no memories elicited) spontaneously linked her current problem to an early memory and rated questions one through six all with the most affirmative rating possible. Even with this case left in the data analysis, there are some interesting results. Table 3.1 gives the mean ratings for each item by both groups.

Table 3.1 Mean Ratings on Client Satisfaction Index Items

Items	1	2	3	4	5	6
Early memory	7.33	7.75	7.33	8.66	7.00	7.00
Control	8.25	7.66	8.58	9.17	6.83	8.25

The control group felt more satisfied, and comfortable with the counselor, and more accepted by the counselor. This group also felt the session was more pleasant. However, the ratings indicate that the group recalling early memories felt that they understood their problem more clearly and felt that discussing the problem was slightly more helpful than the control group reported. The responses to question ten show that only two students indicated that disclosing the early memories was "not really helpful." These results suggest that although the control group felt more comfortable they also felt less helped, whereas the eliciting of the memories made the experimental group on the whole feel less comfortable but more helped. It appears that for some students, satisfaction is more associated with comfort and acceptance than it is with feeling helped and gaining in self-understanding. Of course, unless a therapist has had previous psychodynamic training, the likelihood of enhancing self-understanding by means of early memories would be decreased. However, if a student can find this process helpful with a therapist going by a brief guide sheet, then sessions with a therapist experienced with the method should certainly be beneficial to students. Now the dilemma becomes how to recognize which student will respond best to attempts at insight and self-understanding and which will respond best to acceptance and a comfortable environment.

The general themes of early memories elicited are presented in Appendix C by subject along with presenting problem and identification data. Examining the differences between the clients who felt it was helpful to recall the memories and those who did not shows that subjects 1 and 12, who found the procedure least helpful (question 10), were the youngest students (18 years old) and were passive-dependent females who felt helpless as evidenced by the presenting concern and the

memories described. They used the defense of denial against
feelings of aggression and reproach toward parental figures
despite memories to which the obvious emotional response
would be anger. These students also manifested problems of
depression and poor self-management. Next, the clients who
were unsure as to the value of describing the early memories
(subjects 3 and 6) were also among the younger clients, and
they appeared to have a need to maintain a picture of "goodness" regarding their family relationships as reflected in
the manifest content of the early memories, despite material
they offered suggesting the contrary. The denial of anger
and reproach was more thinly veiled in this group which
presented with concerns having to do with test taking and
study problems. In contradistinction, a review of the group
responding favorably to the recalling of early memories
reveals that these subjects (2, 4, 5, 7, 8, 9, and 11) were
more likely to be older, and to present problems that were
articulated in interpersonal terms if they were male or in
terms of anxiety and "insecurity" if they were female. These
students more easily associated the anger and reproach felt
toward their parents with their present playing out of conflicts.

Thus, it appears that students who are older and have
problems of an interpersonal nature, if they are male, or
problems associated with anxiety or insecurity, if female,
respond better to the eliciting of early memories than do
more depressed, passive-dependent, younger students, who
utilize denial concerning aggressive feelings within themselves or others. The crucial variables here are probably
the passive-dependent personality type and the defense of
denial, particularly around feelings of anger and reproach.
Finally, five of the six subjects who felt the early memories
were "somewhat helpful," "not really helpful," or were unsure
about their value came to the counseling center at the
insistence of a professor while the students themselves were
mildly resistant to coming. Only one of the six subjects
who responded favorably to the early memory eliciting was
urged to come by a third party. It is understandable that
the less-motivated clients did not respond as well to the
treatment, especially considering how the use of early memories focuses on core conflicts that the less-motivated clients would neither desire to examine nor to resolve.

The scale ratings show subjects 9 and 10 rating the
experience the lowest although they indicated that the recalling of early memories was "somewhat" and "partially" helpful
in response to question 10. Both of these students revealed
situations of hostile-dependency in their early memories and
maintained a passive stance in response to their current difficulties coupled with a primitive self-destructive orality
manifested by the abuse of alcohol and food. These individ-

uals were in all likelihood the most disturbed students in the group with respect to ego strength and self-mastery deficits.

Not surprisingly, the students who later reported the memories to be helpful were able to connect their feelings and/or interpersonal behavior in the memories to their present situation. Subject 2 expressed that she felt as if she were still looking for the parents she never had and hence felt insecure. Subject 4 related that the early memories of women leaving him added to his present lack of trust in women and to his expectation that he would be left. Subject 5 connected his early feelings of dependency to his parents' passivity and his wish to be taken care of. Subject 7 felt her wish to be taken care of by her father was related to "blanking out." However, she did not consider aloud the possibilities involving resentment. Subject 8 saw the pattern of preferring to be alone in his memories, as well as at the present time. Subject 9 realized that his negative attention-seeking behavior (for example, milk spilling) continued to be acted out in his drunken rages. Subject 11 was able to see the reenactment of early feelings of incompetency, boredom, and passivity. To the trained observer there were relationships, but perhaps less obvious, between the other subjects' early memories and their present feelings.

Finally, the data from students supported the observation by all of the therapists that the eliciting of early memories was helpful as an intervention for some students but not for others. However, the therapists agreed that it was always beneficial in gaining a more in-depth understanding of the student diagnostically. (It is most likely that this method of assessment gathers psychodynamic material in a much more personal way than a Rorschach or TAT.)

In summary, the findings of this study are consistent with the findings in Chapter 9 regarding what works best with whom and when. Therefore, although the total number of subjects in this preliminary investigation is small, some hypotheses can be made concerning the use of eliciting early memories in the initial phase of counseling or psychotherapy.

Those who will feel helped by this form of treatment are likely to be: older students who come free of coercion, do not have entrenched passive-dependent coping styles, present primarily with insecurity or anxiety if female and interpersonal problems if male, do not have gross ego deficiencies resulting in primitive, impulsive forms of acting out, and who are able in the treatment procedure to relate their feelings or behavior in the memories to their current feelings or behavior.

INSTRUCTIONS TO COUNSELORS

The Significance of Early Memories

The point of interest here is that early memories are frequently diagnostic of one's interpersonal style and self-concept.

The memory stands out as a representation of how we see ourselves in relation to others and the environment and often the scene depicted is a scenario repeated throughout life and may be integrally related to the client's present problem situation. Thus the client may come to see that his present problem is not completely situational but related to a long-standing cognitive set reflected in the early memory.

Procedure for Clients Getting Early Memories Treatment

(1) Get permission to *tape*. Then go on with session as usual.

(2) After this, about 20 minutes into the session, at a comfortable point ask:

"In order to get a better understanding of you as a person, I wonder if you could share your *earliest memory* with me--the earliest scene you can visualize in your mind's eye, whichever one strikes you first. Describe the scene in as much *detail* as possible."
Then get his *next earliest memory too*. It's important to get *two* from each client in this treatment condition.

After allowing time for sufficient elaboration you may want to find out any of the following not offered:

How old was the client in the memories?
Where is the setting?
Who else is in the scene?
What did the client do in the scene?
What was done to the client?
How does the client feel about himself, others, and the environment in the scene?
How do others feel?
What sense modality is primary (e.g., smell, taste)?
What's the outcome?

(3) Then when it feels comfortable ask:

"Do you see any relation between how you acted and felt in the early memories and how you've acted and felt recently?"

(4) At the end of the session say: "I'd appreciate it if you'd fill this *Client Satisfaction Index* out for me to help in evaluating our services and leave it with the secretary. Thanks." (Further questions may be answered after CSI is turned in.)

Procedure for Control (No Memories) Clients

(1) Get permission to *tape*. Then go on with session as usual.

(2) At the end ask:

"I'd appreciate it if you'd fill this *Client Satisfaction Index* out for me to help in evaluating our services and leave it with the secretary. Thanks."

APPENDIX B

CLIENT SATISFACTION INDEX

(1) I feel satisfied with the session.

       1   2   3   4   5   6   7   8   9   10

Not at all Somewhat Moderately Quite Extremely

(2) Discussing the problem was helpful to me.

       1   2   3   4   5   6   7   8   9   10

Not at all Somewhat Moderately Quite Extremely

(3) I felt comfortable with the counselor.

       1   2   3   4   5   6   7   8   9   10

Not at all Somewhat Moderately Quite Extremely

(4) I felt the counselor accepted me as an individual.

       1   2   3   4   5   6   7   8   9   10

Not at all Somewhat Moderately Quite Extremely

(5) I understand my problem more clearly as a result of the session.

       1   2   3   4   5   6   7   8   9   10

Not at all Somewhat Moderately Quite Extremely

(6) The session was:

       1   2   3   4   5   6   7   8   9   10

    Unpleasant   Pleasant   Very Pleasant

(7) What part of the session was most helpful?

(8) What part was least helpful?

(9) What was it like describing your early memories?

(10) Was it helpful in understanding your problem?

GENERAL THEMES OF EARLY MEMORIES BY SUBJECT
AND PRESENTING PROBLEM

Subject	Early Memory Themes	Presenting Problem and Identification Data
1	a. Mother dresses her up very "cutesy" and peers at school make fun of her (age 5).	Depression. She is a freshman and an only child.
	b. The whole class was given a punishment which consisted of looking up the definitions of many words. The client and her parents stayed up very late working on it together (age 9).	
2	a. In the crib on Halloween "in your own little world" someone with a Mickey Mouse mask looked in through the window and terrified her (age 2).	Chronic insecurity. She is the mother of two children and came back to school at age 27 to become a nurse.
	b. After staying with her grandparents for quite a while her mother came to "reclaim" her. The client "threw a fit" as she did not want to leave what felt like her "real home." "Mom's never been there . . . it feels like I had no parents . . . Mom said Dad wouldn't have left her if she hadn't had children" (age 2).	
3	a. Falling down, playing alone and cutting her chin.	Blanking on exams. She is the youngest child and a sophomore.
	b. Again falling down and cutting her chin while running to show parents her caterpillar collec-	

Appendix C (continued)

Subject	Early Memory Themes	Presenting Problem and Identification Data
	tion as the parents were driving out the driveway to a party. The client remembers this as a happy time (both at age 4 or 5).	
4	a. Stepmother's death, "what a time to die, just as I was getting this award" (age 9).	Problems with trusting women not to leave him. He is a senior.
	b. Dad asked him to meet his new wife after mother died (age 7).	
5	a. Fourth birthday party-- very happy.	Trouble getting active in job search. He is a 24-year-old gratuate student.
	b. Sixth birthday party, a friend broke his toy lawn mower. He was angry at the friend and his mother for not taking care of him.	
6	a. A parade on the Fourth of July, he is happy with his family and friends (age 4).	Total lack of interest in his work and problems relating to his authoritarian father. He is a 20-year-old undergraduate.
	b. Playing in the yard with his father, very happy (age 4).	
7	a. Flushing the alarm clock from her parents' bedroom down the toilet.	Blanking on tests. She is an only child and a sophomore.
	b. Dad coming home from a long time away, very happy (unsure of age, but both are before age 5).	
8	a. Joy of playing in the water alone while strangers watched (age 3).	Feels "closed in on" in close relationships.

b. Playing ball alone, "a solitary activity" (age 4).

He is a 28-year-old graduate student.

9 a. Crying in his mother's lap after watching a bird on a television cartoon get killed (age 2).

b. Spilling milk in his high chair (acknowledged later that it was to get attention from mother) (age 2).

Anxiety due to not being able to have roommate's girlfriend or to get close to any other women, deals with anxiety by getting drunk and angry. He is a 21-year-old junior.

10 a. Playing with her friends who went home to watch television. She could not go with them or watch at home as her family had no television. The client felt angry.

Seemed unable to begin her thesis, also moderate anxiety and depression.

b. In the hospital to have tonsils removed, grandfather was with her but mother was absent . . . "Mother was pregnant . . . Mother was never there" (age 4).

She is a 25-year-old graduate student in nursing and quite overweight.

11 a. Playing in the snow with siblings, losing her sled in the snow and being afraid that she will not be able to find it, feeling bored watching others play.

Anxiety stemming from fears of not being able to succeed on her own or to be independent. She is a 21-year-old junior.

b. Sitting at home in the living room watching her sister and parents all engage in some crafts or work while she felt "out of it" (age 3).

12 a. "Running to meet Dad after work and sitting on a big pipe near a pit, very happy."

b. "Going to a speech therapist, not liking it" (age 5).

Difficulty organizing her time to study. She is an 18-year-old freshman, is depressed, passive, and interacts in a child-like manner.

REFERENCES

Adcock, N. "Early Memories and Sex Differences." *New Zealand Psychologist* 4 (1975):30-34.

Adler, A. "The Significance of Early Childhood Recollections." *International Journal of Individual Psychology* 3 (1937): 283-287.

Binder, J. and I. Smokler. "Early Memories: A Technical Aid to Focusing in Time-Limited Dynamic Psychotherapy." *Psychotherapy: Theory, Research and Practice* 17 (1980): 52-62.

Brodsky, P. "The Diagnostic Importance of Early Recollections." *American Journal of Psychotherapy* 6 (1952):484-493.

Burnell, G. and G. Solomon. "Early Memories and Ego Function." *Archives of General Psychiatry* 11 (1964):556-567.

Chess, S. "Utilization of Childhood Memories in Psychoanalytic Therapy." *Journal of Child Psychiatry* 2 (1951):187-193.

Eisenstein, V. and R. Ryerson. "The Psychodynamic Significance of the First Conscious Memory." *Bulletin of the Menninger Clinic* 15 (1951):213-220.

Ferguson, E. "The Use of Early Recollections for Assessing Life Style and Diagnosing Psychopathology." *Journal of Projective Techniques and Personality Assessment* 28 (1964): 403-412.

Freud, S. "Screen Memories." In *Collected Papers, Vol. 5.* London: Hogarth Press, 1950. Pp. 47-69.

Gellert, S. "How to Reach Early Scenes and Decisions by Dream Work." *Transactional Analysis Journal* 6 (1976):144-146.

Goulding, M. and R. Goulding. *Changing Lives Through Redecision Therapy.* New York: Brunner-Mazel, 1979.

Greve, B. "Protocol Fantasy and Early Decision." *Transactional Analysis Journal* 6 (1976):46-60.

Langs, R. "Earliest Memories and Personality: A Predictive Study." *Archives of General Psychiatry* 12 (1965):379-390.

Langs, R., M. Rothenberg, J. Fishman, and M. Reiser. "A Method for the Clinical and Theoretical Study of the Earliest Memory." *Archives of General Psychiatry* 3 (1960):523-534.

Levy, J. "Early Memories: Theoretical Aspects and Applica-
    tions." *Journal of Projective Techniques and Personality
    Assessment* 29 (1965):281-291.

Lieberman, M. "Childhood Memories as a Projective Test."
    Journal of Projective Techniques 21 (1957):32-36.

Mayman, M. "Early Memories and Character Structure." *Journal
    of Projective Techniques and Personality Assessment* 32
    (1968):303-316.

Mayman, M. and M. Faris. "Early Memories as Expressions of
    Relationship Paradigms." *American Journal of Orthopsychi-
    atry* 30 (1970):507-520.

Saul, L., T. Snyder, and A. Sheppard. "On Earliest Memories."
    Psychoanalytic Quarterly 26 (1956):228-237.

4

Treating the Grieving Student

Elinor T. Roy

The experience of coping with death and mourning is common for university students. By graduation, approximately 10 percent of this population has lost one parent to death, with death of a father twice as common as death of a mother (Werner & Jones 1979). In addition to the deaths or terminal illnesses of parents, students often face the death of grandparents as well. Other losses, although certainly less frequent, include those of friends, usually by automobile accident or by suicide. Because these events are often the students' first significant encounters with death, they generally have limited experiences or coping skills on which to rely.

However, grieving also occurs after other losses. In a college community, students frequently experience the loss of relationships. LaGrand (1981), in one of the few studies of loss reactions in college and university students, asked over 1,000 students to report recent major losses. Of the respondents, 77 percent reported losses of significant others by death, by end of friendship or love relationship, by parental divorce, or by the students' own divorce. Another sense of loss frequent in this population occurs as a result of abortion.

As with all stressful events, the manner in which the loss is perceived determines its significance. Failure in a course, the death of a pet, the loss of a long-time goal, or the suspension of a roommate from school may be viewed as insignificant by some, but may have immense impact on others. While grief therapy most commonly looks at the process of mourning resulting from the death of a loved one, the counselor or therapist in a university setting may also frequently encounter grief reactions to other types of losses and should approach the treatment in a similar manner. This chapter describes a treatment process for goal-oriented, time-limited grief therapy primarily for normal grief reactions. However, for some students with good ego strength, these techniques may be appropriate for work with abnormal grief reactions as well.

A DEVELOPMENTAL CONTEXT

In a university counseling center, issues of loss and mourning must be considered in relation to the period of late adolescence and young adulthood. The developmental tasks of this age group are as follows:

1. developing autonomy, changing from relationships of dependence to independence;
2. dealing with authority;
3. learning to deal with ambiguity and ambivalence;
4. developing a capacity for intimacy;
5. developing a mature sexuality and solidifying a sexual identity;
6. learning to effectively manage emotions;
7. clarifying a sense of purpose with a formulation of life plans and vocation;
8. developing a personal value system; and
9. attaining a sense of adequacy and competence (Chickering 1972, Farnsworth 1966).

Normal development for most students does not proceed smoothly. At any stage, a crisis may interfere with growth and reduce opportunities for personal fulfillment. Progress through any or all of these stages might be affected by a significant loss, such as the death of a parent.

Developing Autonomy

The most difficult task of adolescence is to relinquish the security that is maintained by dependence on parents. Achieving independence entails a reworking of the earlier process of separation/individuation. Much has been written about the mourning process involved in this loss of security. Grief is also a form of separation reaction. Thus, the normal developmental task becomes complicated when a parent dies. There is a concomitant threat to identity and a loss of the way the student views and defines her/himself. Some of the effects of such a loss of security can be seen in the example of Edie, a sophomore who had been appropriately separating from her family and becoming increasingly independent. After her father's death she returned to a helpless and dependent role with both her family and her boyfriend. Her boyfriend's complaints about her clinging brought her to our service, obviously regressed and in need of support.

Dealing with Authority

The issue here is one of power, specifically, how students deal with their own power and the power of others. The relationships of young adults with persons in authority are, to some extent, reflections of their relationships with adult family members. Thus, loss of such an individual may complicate the task of dealing with authority figures. Many college students are in the midst of an "adolescent rebellion" that requires having someone to rebel against. The removal of this source of stability may leave the student so angry as to become globally rebellious or feeling so guilty about prior rebellion as to withdraw the questioning of authority that is necessary in order to develop autonomy.

Learning to Deal with Ambiguity

The student is learning to recognize that the world is not just black and white, but also consists of shades of gray. The task is to reckon with idealism that is in conflict with reality. The inherent ambivalence in the grief process with its mixture of feelings such as sadness, anger, and guilt, may strain the not yet developed tolerance for ambivalence and ambiguity. This dilemma is exemplified by Ann, a college freshman whose father committed suicide shortly before she entered school. She was unable to begin reconciling her rage at him for abandoning the family with her awareness of the pain that he was in before his death until she spent a substantial amount of time and effort in therapy.

Developing a Capacity for Intimacy and a Mature Sexuality

There is a need to replace familial closeness with new relationships and to balance risk taking with tolerance for being vulnerable. After a major loss, however, there may be a desire to withdraw emotionally. The fear of a future loss may make it more difficult to enter and sustain a loving relationship. The case of Jenny illustrates this.

Jenny came to Counseling and Psychological Services after a series of brief relationships with men, all of which she had quickly ended. Although she liked and respected these young men, she found herself retreating emotionally and sexually

time after time. It became apparent that she was being influenced by her parents' divorce, which had taken place
several years earlier. Her father had left his wife and
children, moved to the West Coast with a new wife and her
family, and severed most ties with his own children. Jenny's
motto had unconsciously become, "Don't get close to men or
trust them. Leave them before they can leave you."

Managing Emotions

This task involves learning to integrate emotions with
behavior and decision making. During grieving students are
often flooded with affect that previous methods of handling
their emotions are no longer adequate. They may then become
frightened and think they are "going crazy." This is particularly true when their friends are unable, due to inexperi-
ence, to validate their new, more intense feelings.

Clarifying Purpose

This task entails making life plans for the future and
setting priorities in a framework that integrates vocational,
avocational, and recreational interests. Loss, particularly
of a parent, may make it more difficult to identify with that
parent in a positive manner and to choose a similar career.
Conversely, the loss may cause the student to abandon his/her
own plans and engage in an unhealthy identification by adoption of some aspect of the deceased's behavior. This is an
attempt to hold on to the deceased. An example is the art
student who feels compelled to change his career path in
order to follow that of his scientist father. Often, too,
we see students who have lost a long term goal. For example,
students who are rejected by medical school after pursuing
that goal for years, and are now grieving the loss of that
dream, and feeling a lack of purpose and direction.

Developing a Personal Value System

As the student achieves increasing independence, s/he
must clarify and personalize beliefs to develop a source of
inner guidance for behavior. Adolescence is usually a time
of questioning formerly held beliefs, but sudden losses can
cause disarray in forming the framework for a personal value
system.
For example, Hannah was a student whose mother was terminally ill with uterine cancer. Hannah's presenting complaint was that she was having difficulty reconciling her

promiscuity with her previously held attitudes toward sexuality. The anticipated loss had so overwhelmed her that Hannah's usual values and decision making were disrupted. She then sought caring and proof of her adequacy through sexual acting out.

Attaining Competence

The student is beginning to see her/himself as an adult and wishes to be seen by others in this way. The task is to find security and to develop feelings of adequacy in intellectual, physical, vocational, and interpersonal areas. The grieving student may feel out of control. Feelings of adequacy and competence are compromised by the student's feeling unable to cope with the loss. The two pitfalls associated with this task are regressing into a childlike role or being thrust prematurely into an adult role. An example of the latter is found in a freshman who after the death of his father felt pressured to leave school and return home to become "the man of the family."

In helping our students work through their grief experiences, it is of utmost importance to examine their mourning in the context of the normal developmental tasks they are also facing. In addition, the counselor needs an understanding of the normal grieving process in order to be able to differentiate between normal and abnormal grief during the evaluation process.

THE EXPERIENCE OF NORMAL GRIEF

Uncomplicated (normal) grief runs a consistent, predictable course. The acute phase of normal grief typically lasts six to eight weeks, with symptoms almost always similar to those of depression. They include sadness, sleep difficulty, appetite disturbance, weight loss, general loss of interest, and difficulty in concentration. In about half of all bereaved persons, these symptoms continue on an intermittent basis throughout the first year following the loss and some emotional reactions may continue for several years (Parkes 1972).

In his classic paper, "The Symptomatology and Management of Acute Grief," Lindemann (1944) described pathognomonic characteristics of normal or acute grief:

1. Somatic or bodily distress.
2. Preoccupation with the image of the deceased.
3. Guilt regarding the deceased or the circumstances surrounding the death.

4. Hostile reactions.
5. The inability to function as before the loss.
6. The development of traits of the deceased
   in the bereaved person's behavior.

During grief, phenomena occur that would ordinarily signal pathology or the loss of reality testing. Counselors should be aware that almost half of all bereaved persons report some form of hallucination or "sense of the presence" of the deceased (Rees 1975; Clayton et al. 1968). Thus, counselors should not view such reports from clients as necessarily pathologic. Having this understanding can also enable counselors to give reassurance to students who understandably fear "going crazy."

DIAGNOSIS AND ASSESSMENT

Accurate recognition and assessment of grief can be problematic. First, students with major losses often present with vague complaints and may not volunteer information on death or loss since they do not see a direct correlation between their current problems and loss. Because of this, a "loss history" is a very important part of an intake procedure and should not be overlooked. The therapist needs to look not only for current losses, but also for old, unresolved loss experiences, sometimes signaled by anniversary reactions. The "hidden loss syndrome" may include "taboo" experiences such as a rape or an abortion that has not been previously revealed.

Another problem for counselors is that grief reactions can be misdiagnosed as depression, since there are many similarities between the two conditions. In both presentations, there are symptoms of sleep and appetite disturbance and strong feelings of sadness. Worden (1982) notes that in grief reactions, however, the client will not usually experience the loss of self-esteem that s/he would in depression. The feelings of guilt also differ. In grief, guilt is typically connected to only one phase of the loss as opposed to the overall sense of culpability found in depression.

Once the therapist has ascertained that a grief reaction is present, it becomes necessary to decide if the presentation is normal grief as previously described or abnormal grief.

ABNORMAL GRIEF

Time and intensity are used to differentiate abnormal or unresolved grief from normal grief. Melges and DeMaso (1980)

describe abnormal grief as "too little grieving soon after
the loss or too much grieving too long after the loss or
both." The bereaved seems tied to the past, and limited in
ability to relate to the present or future, and feels that
no amount of time will ever heal the loss.

The counselor may find three different types of pathologic grief reactions (Sustento 1969):

1. There may be absence of emotion in an effort to avoid
the intense pain of grief. The student may experience deper-
sonalization or complain of being "foggy." Often, there is
an inability to see the connection between current discomfort
and the loss.

2. Unusually prolonged grief reactions may become self-
perpetuating. Idealization of the deceased to instant saint-
hood allows unpleasant aspects of the relationship to remain
repressed and prevents the working through of the grief process.

3. Exaggerated grief may be due to feelings of guilt and
the need for punishment. For example, Sam, whose father had
died ten years earlier, experienced extraordinary guilt and
grief because he felt the financial situation of their blue
collar family improved after the death as a result of subsequent life insurance payments and Social Security benefits
that paid for Sam's education. Yet another student, Linda,
was aware of masochistic tendencies that seemed related to
unresolved grief for her father who had died during her early
childhood. She experienced much guilt over having wished
that he would die during his prolonged illness and, with the
magical thinking typical of early childhood, felt from that
point onward she was somehow responsible for his death. The
need for punishment generated by these feelings seemed to
lead to her characteristic masochistic style.

It should be noted that most abnormal or unresolved grief
reactions are not suitable for brief, crisis-oriented treatment. Generally, persons with such longstanding or problematic grief require longer-term therapy. However, there are
exceptions, and given the age and ego strength of many college
students, there are many students with abnormal grief reactions who can and do profit from brief grief therapy lasting
from 8 to 14 sessions.

The third area of assessment that will help to determine
the length and type of counseling required is an examination
of the context in which the reaction to loss is occurring.
The therapist needs to evaluate the student's usual coping
skills. How are anxiety and depression managed? How have
past losses been handled? Attention should be paid to ego
strength and defense mechanisms and how they have been
affected by the loss as well as any noticeable dysfunction

in feelings, thoughts, or behavior. As previously discussed, a developmental framework is helpful in assessment. Considerations might include where the student is regarding the developmental tasks as well as what psychosocial crises may coincide with or be exacerbated by the reaction to loss. A determination should be made of the nature of the relationship or family situation before the loss. The counselor should also attempt to evaluate social supports. How have family, friends, and the campus community responded to the student? If the student is devoutly religious, does it appear that religious beliefs will be an aid to the grief work, or will the beliefs increase conflict and thus be a deterrent to the healing process? For example, consider the Roman Catholic student who cannot bear the religious conflict and resultant guilt following her abortion. A final and important part of the assessment is to determine by direct and specific inquiry whether the client is suicidal.

In addition to normal and abnormal grief, students may present with yet another form of grief reaction, specifically, a concern about an impending loss, or anticipatory grief. Examples of this may be found in response to terminally ill family members or friends, the impending loss of a love relationship, the student's own or a parental divorce, or an unplanned pregnancy and preabortion concerns. It is the task of the therapist to assist the student in understanding that such situations may arouse anticipatory grief and to help the student understand the current experience and feelings in that light. The grieving process and grief counseling are virtually the same with regard to anticipatory grief with other types of loss but much of the emphasis is on the future rather than the past.

THE TASKS OF MOURNING

It is helpful for both client and therapist to have an understanding of the tasks of the mourning process. Viewing grief work as a series of tasks is similar to the concept of "developmental tasks" frequently utilized by college counselors. The incompletion of grief tasks can impair future growth and development while their completion can foster growth and increased autonomy. This task approach suggests that the mourner needs to assume an active stance to do something about the situation. This orientation implies, too, that mourning can be affected by intervention. Although the grief tasks may seem overwhelming to the mourner, with the help of a therapist, hope becomes accessible as an antidote for the impotence that most mourners feel. Worden (1982) has outlined four tasks.

Task I: To Accept the Reality of the Loss

Following the loss, the bereaved feels shock and dis-
belief that such an irreversible loss could occur. These
feelings are adaptive responses that allow the person time
to mobilize defenses against affect that could overwhelm.
During this period there is a struggle with denial that can
take many forms, including minimizing the loss ("We weren't
really that close," "He was never the father I wanted"), or
"selective forgetting." Students may block the image or even
the reality of the person from mind.

Task II: To Experience the Pain of Grief

The theory of grief work presupposes that pain must be
acknowledged and worked through or it will manifest itself
through another symptom or behavior. Persons who find it
difficult to experience pain may attempt to avoid painful
fellings by intellectualizing, idealizing the dead, or shun-
ning reminders of the deceased.

Task III: To Adjust to an Environment
in Which the Deceased Is Missing

The adjustment to a different environment depends on the
relationship between the bereaved and the deceased and the
diverse roles the deceased played. This adjustment may
involve the bereaved taking on roles previously assumed by
the deceased and, thus, make the acquisition of new skills a
necessity. Survivors must struggle to face up to new responsibilities rather than submitting to feelings of helplessness
and a desire to withdraw. One part of this task is to reframe
the loss so that the growth-related aspects can be realized.

Task IV: To Withdraw Emotional Energy and
Reinvest It in Another Relationship

This final task involves achieving an emotional withdrawal
from the deceased person so that energy can be devoted to other relationships. Some people choose to hold on to the past
rather than opening up their lives to new possibilities.
Others find the experience of loss so difficult that they
decide to avoid the risk of another loss by not getting involved again. For many, this is the most difficult task and
may result in the feeling that they are "stuck." It may also
take some time to perform this task (Worden 1982). One student whose father had died while she was in high school wrote

home from college, "I have just realized that it's okay to
go on with my life now, to have fun and date and that fact
doesn't mean I love Dad less" (Worden 1982).

The process of mourning is considered complete when these
tasks are finished and the survivor has returned to the former level of functioning with the feelings of intense pain
gone. Although the time frame varies greatly with the individual, resolution after the loss of a close relationship
does not usually occur for a year or two. One of the counselor's most important tasks in grief counseling is to educate clients that mourning is a long-term process.

EXTERNAL AND INTERNAL FACTORS
INHIBITING MOURNING

In preparing to assist students in the grief process,
therapists also need to understand that there are a number of
external and internal factors that may prevent the tasks of
mourning from being successfully completed.

External Factors

One external factor is the expectation that the mourner
engage in "practical" behaviors that are not connected with
the emotions of the loss--for example, arranging to be away
from classes, making travel plans, planning the funeral, and
so on. A second external factor is the cultural and social
constraint put on the display of grief. Value is often
placed on a show of "strength" as opposed to "weak" or
"childish" overt weeping and grieving. The young person striving toward adulthood may find this particularly difficult.
Often the bereaved may be forced into the role of supporter
for other mourners. The student may be told, "You must be
the man of the family now," or "Be strong for your mother and
younger sisters." If the student is not seen as the rescuer,
s/he must at least not be perceived as an additional source
of discomfort or trouble.

Other external factors that may inhibit mourning exist
for students who are still adjusting to an unfamiliar environment and have not yet developed a support system. Students
who attend college away from home are separated from the community and support of fellow mourners when the loss occurs in
the home community.

If time away from school (for the funeral) is necessary,
there will be pressures to return and resume academic work
rather quickly or run the risk of losing a term's work. When
the student returns to campus, the environment tends to foster repression and denial. "It's hard to believe it's real

because my life at school goes on as usual. I don't think
it'll really hit me until I'm home for vacation." Students
report that there is generally a noticeable lack of support
from their peers within a few weeks following the loss.
Adolescents and young adults have little information about
grief or experience with it and are not aware of how long
grieving continues or the amount of pain associated with it.
They generally feel awkward and ill at ease in comforting
those who have suffered losses. "My friends don't know what
to say to me about his death so they don't say anything.
They treat me as if it never happened except everything seems
awkward now." The intensity of feelings and the fear of
contagion frighten students as well. A student might think,
"If this can happen to your family, then it could happen in
mine."

Finally, the use of tranquilizers and antidepressants
sometimes serve to suppress normal grief and anxiety. In
some cases the grief and mourning are "chemically held in
abeyance only to erupt later" (Barry 1973). Therapists need
to ask their clients if they are taking prescribed medication
or are medicating themselves through borrowed or old medications, alcohol, or recreational drug use.

Internal Factors

A number of internal factors may inhibit mourning as
well. Children are often taught to control feelings; in
other words, "Big boys and girls don't cry." This suppres-
sion of feeling may carry over into adolescence and adulthood
and affect how individuals handle loss. There may also be a
fear that feelings will be overwhelming and that expressing
them will be to no avail.

Another factor possibly inhibiting affect concerns
timing. If one can't mourn at the appropriate time, that is,
immediately following the loss, later expression of feeling
may seem inappropriate. If there is a stigma associated with
the loss such as in the case of suicide or abortion, suppres-
sion of feelings may result. Individuals may also feel as
if they have no right to experience relief at the death of
a loved one who has been in pain and suffering from a long
illness such as cancer.

Anger or ambivalence may also block mourning. Feelings
of being abandoned by the deceased or conflicting feelings
about past experiences may then be covered over by adoration
for the lost person. There is also the admonition, "Don't
speak ill of the dead." As a result, anger is often directed
toward the self or others instead of the deceased and thus
grieving is inhibited. As every new loss reminds one of
previous losses, there may be fears of resurrecting old con-

flicts if feelings of sadness are allowed in the current situation. Finally, overidentification with the deceased may also prevent mourning. This can prompt concern that one may give up oneself by giving up the deceased.

Some other factors blocking expression of the emotions binding the bereaved to the deceased are seen less often, but are still present in the college population. They include: "contracts" with the deceased ("I won't leave you as you left me"); secrets or unfinished business ("I'll keep you alive to forgive me"); and finally, the secondary gain found in remaining grief stricken. This is most frequently seen in very dependent persons who wish to find a way of escaping from responsibilities (Melges & DeMaso 1980).

GRIEF THERAPY

The goal of grief therapy is to facilitate the mourning tasks of normal grief so that the bereavement process can proceed toward a successful "conclusion" or, in grief that is absent, prolonged, delayed, or excessive, to identify and resolve those conflicts that prevent the successful accomplishment of the mourning tasks. Grief work is "a kind of housecleaning in which the relationship of the griever to the lost object in all its ambivalence is relived and emotionally reevaluated bit by bit so that emotional detachment can finally be achieved" (Barry 1981). In addition to facilitating normal and anticipatory grief and dealing with unresolved grief, the therapist's task is to help the student learn about the loss process so that there is preparation for inevitable future losses.

Whether normal or abnormal, grief is stressful. Bereaved clients frequently present in crisis and if grief work is viewed in relation to a crisis intervention model, one assumes that individuals are particularly amenable to help at that time. Lydia Rapoport (1965) suggests, "a little help, rationally directed and purposefully focused at a strategic time is more effective than more extreme help given at a period of less emotional accessibility." If the initial assessment establishes a grief issue as central, then the therapist's first tasks are: to form an alliance, to provide information about the grief process, and to set the treatment contract.

A strong therapeutic alliance is crucial in grief work since the goal of treatment is to facilitate conflict resolution which might require the client to experience feelings that previously have been avoided. As Worden (1982) states, "The therapist provides the social support system necessary for all successful grief work and essentially gives the patient permission to grieve, permission which the patient, in his or her previous social environment, was not granted."

Because of the nature of treatment and because the bereaved person often feels helpless, the therapist should
demonstrate expert authority by being direct. Helping the
client to define the issue as a grief reaction is one of the
counselor's first tasks, followed by providing information
about the process of grief work. This information should
include facts about the symptoms of grief, factors that may
influence or inhibit mourning and the tasks of mourning.
The therapist explains that grief is a painful process, and
in some sense it is never completely finished, but by working through and ventilating feelings, there is relief. Such
information helps the student develop a causal understanding
of the pain. Many students have feared they were "going
crazy" because of the intensity of their feelings and because
previous coping skills were found to be ineffectual. This
is particularly true if the client has experienced the dis-
turbing "sense of the presence of the deceased" or hallucinations. To be told that this is not pathological but normal
greatly allays anxiety.

Partializing the problem by assessing the remaining
mourning tasks helps to alleviate some of the client's helplessness as well. The therapist explains that the counseling
process will include a review of the relationship with the
deceased and the various feelings that the client may have
with the specific understanding that the client will determine the pace of the work based on personal comfort. The
therapist acknowledges and recognizes the difficulty in opening up feelings about a loss, but states the necessity of
sharing the grief in order to produce an emotional catharsis
and reduce the tension that has been immobilizing the client.
The emphasis, too, is on the fact that this is a process
which can provide relief. The client is reassured that grief
therapy is effective if s/he can invest in the work with the
expectation of both subjective relief and behavioral change.
The bereaved's hopelessness is counteracted by the counselor's expression of confidence in the student's capacity to
resolve the grief. Hope is ego supportive in beginning the
process of grief resolution.

Grief therapy is typically a time-limited treatment,
usually requiring no more than eight to ten sessions. This
treatment program fits well with the time constraints of the
usual academic term and the brief therapy model of most
counseling centers. As with other forms of short-term treatment, the therapy needs to be highly focused and goal oriented. Although the counselor should use the constraint of
time to provide structure and limits, it is important to
remain flexible. The grieving client feels out of control
and this can be of particular concern to adolescents and
young adults for whom autonomy and control issues are central. It is helpful, if the therapist's schedule permits, to

let the student set the timing of the second visit, perhaps by offering other times in the same week. In addition to reinforcing the student's control, this flexibility and accessibility to the therapist also aids in developing the therapeutic alliance.

Clients generally return for subsequent sessions willing to work but wary of eliciting the pain that they now know to be a part of the healing process. The therapist may need to remind the student that s/he is in control of the pace of the grief work.

The next phase of treatment includes the tasks of reviewing the relationship, facing the facts of the actual loss, expressing feelings, learning new skills, reworking and reframing the loss, and saying a final goodbye. This part of treatment begins with reviewing the relationship with the lost person and the therapist prescribing "dosages of reminiscences." Clients might be encouraged to bring in a photo of the deceased. Individuals generally feel more comfortable beginning with positive memories about the relationship such as the person's qualities and characteristics, and memories of activities and times shared. Spending a good deal of time in these early sessions reviewing enjoyable memories serves several purposes. First, it develops a foundation of positive memories that will provide balance for later exploration of the more negative aspects. Second, the therapist is receiving additional information about the basis of the attachment, the strength and security the relationship provided, and clues regarding more ambivalent feelings (Worden 1982). Third, the interest and supportive environment supplied by the counselor help to further forge the therapeutic alliance.

Early in the process of treatment it is helpful to deal with the facts about the actual loss and the circumstances surrounding it. Questions regarding a death might include: "Where were you and how did you learn of it? How did the death occur? What was the funeral or service like?" Answering these questions aids the client in accepting and dealing with the reality and finality of the loss and also provides useful information for the therapist about some of the blocks to mourning that may have occurred. As these events are reviewed often throughout treatment, they typically become more detailed and more closely linked with affect. Positive verbal reinforcement is given for completing these, as well as other steps of the grief work.

Gradually and gently the counselor leads into the more ambivalent feelings by granting permission for and legitimizing the student's negative feelings, just as was done with the positive ones. The counselor might say, "All relationships have minuses as well as pluses. I wonder if you could tell me about some of the difficult or less satisfying aspects of this relationship?" Another might say, "We've

discussed many of the things you've missed about this relationship, what don't you miss?" If the client finds this
difficult, the counselor should pursue why it is so difficult
to recall feelings that are not positive. The counselor
should give reassurance concerning the universality of ambivalence and the need for such feelings to occur in order to
promote the identification and expression of feelings and
memories concerning disappointment, hurt, guilt, and anger.
If the therapist and the student succeed in dealing with the
ambivalence, then it can help in mastering the developmental
task of tolerating ambiguity in a more global way.

Students often feel anger, particularly in reaction to
being left. Anger that is not focused on the deceased may
either be displaced or be turned inward and felt as depression or decreased self-esteem. The counselor should always
check out the possibility of suicidal ideation. Worden
(1982) notes, "Suicidal thoughts do not always represent
retroflected anger. They can also come from a desire to re-
join the deceased." (For a useful guide to the evaluation
of suicide potential, see C. Margolin's "Evaluating Suicide
Potential in the Emergency Department," *Journal of Emergency
Nursing* Vol. 3, 1977.)

Students who had previously tended to view their world
in an idealized way often find their illusions shattered by
a loss. This may result in anger toward God. Religious
doctrines and traditional morality that already may have been
under scrutiny now may become even more suspect. If there
are a number of such existential or religious questions or
fears about feelings of anger toward God, it is often beneficial to refer to a known sympathetic member of the clergy for
adjunctive sessions. Also, many students find helpful Kushner's book, *When Bad Things Happen to Good People* (1981).

Guilt is another feeling that is almost universal. Much
guilt is irrational and can often be traced to the circumstances around the death, particularly an unsatisfactory or
angry last interaction. Young adults can be quite grandiose
in their beliefs and need help in whittling this culpability
down to reasonable size. The guilt may take two forms.
First, reasonable guilt may exist if a parent dies after an
adolescent has been rebelliously acting out. The therapist
needs to help the adolescent understand the universality of
separation/individuation while also helping the student to
take responsibility for the acting out behavior. Second,
irrational guilt may exist and must be examined through reality testing, with the student being "given permission" for
self forgiveness concerning perceived sins of omission or
commission.

Feelings of anxiety and helplessness are also rampant in
persons with a recent loss. Adolescents and young adults
may regress because their achievement of autonomy may be rela-

tively recent and fragile. Often, too, when individuals are
most in need of support they are least able to seek it.
Helping students utilize the support system that is available
to them is beneficial. This system might include resident
advisors, deans, and campus clergy, as well as family and
friends.

Problem solving, developing new skills, and exploring
and rehearsing new familiar or social roles necessitated by
the loss are ways of counteracting the impotence felt in
adjusting to life without the deceased. Clients need help,
too, in understanding the impact of the stress caused by the
loss and subsequent changes in their lives. Some students
will wish to institute major changes, such as transferring
or dropping out of school, as ways of relieving the pain they
feel. For some students, such as the foreign exchange student who needs the support from extended family and a familiar culture, this may be the most appropriate move. For
others, it may be premature or a desire to escape. The task
of the counselor is to help the student sort this out. Other
students may try to reinvest too quickly with a "rebound"
relationship. Engel (1981) warns of problems as well with
the therapeutic relationship. "The counselor helps in the
transition to new relationships and avoids becoming the new
relationship. This is not an easy task." It is important
that the therapist give information on stress management and,
in particular, emphasize the need to minimize life changes
for a time until equilibrium can be restored.

Finally, feelings of sadness need to be expressed. It
is difficult for many clients, particularly young men, to
feel comfortable openly crying, yet this expression of sadness is needed and should be encouraged by the counselor.
The counselor might say, "It must be sad for you to think
about going through life without your fiancé. Is it sad for
you to think about graduation without him?" If the student
still seems blocked, the counselor might explore the cause.
"What makes it hard for you to express how sad you're feeling?" Additionally, counselors should remember that on
occasion it is more appropriate to support the right not to
be sad if the client does not feel sadness; for example,
following the death of a parent with a chronic illness accompanied by much pain, or the death of an abusive parent. Clients often express relief at being given permission to express
whatever they have been suppressing for so long.

As in other forms of therapy, there can be no "cookbook"
approach. The individual needs of the client must be considered. Therapists need to respect the client's defenses
since such defenses may be clues in reevaluating ego strength.
If the therapist senses ego deficits, then pulling back is
appropriate in order not to push the client beyond what will
be comfortably tolerated.

As the student is better able to deal with feelings and the expression of them, it is useful to return in detail to the circumstances of the death and the events following it, such as the wake, sitting shiva, funeral, and so on. At this time the counselor should review what occurred and what the client's feelings were. The following are examples. Jack: "I hated the way I was told about his death. They called and woke me up. I was all alone in my dorm room. It was an awful and long night." Mary Ellen: "The funeral service was so impersonal and artificial. It didn't even seem to relate to her at all." The therapist may offer the opportunity to go back in thought and re-do the event via fantasy the way the client would have wished it to happen. Jack created a scenario in which his family notified his best friend and a college dean so that they would give the news to him. In his fantasy, he was given the support he had longed for and never received. Subsequently he felt able to grieve rather than suppress his feelings as he had done thus far. Mary Ellen creatively designed a memorial service for her mother that was personal and meaningful to her.

This technique of reworking feelings through reconstruction in fantasy allows clients the freedom to mourn in their own way, resume some control, and put these events, now successfully reframed, behind them. Judy often spoke of her memories of her daily walk by the river with her grandmother. Judy did not wish to participate in the ceremony of scattering the ashes, not wanting that to be her final goodbye. She made her fantasy real by actually taking a memorial walk along the river and saying her goodbye in the way she wished.

Final goodbyes are important for all clients in the grieving process. The therapist can help provide an opportunity by asking questions such as: "If you could have the opportunity what would you like to say to ----? What would you tell him/her about what s/he meant to you? Is there unfinished business between you that you'd like to clear up? How would you like to let ---- know what part of him/her you'll always carry with you?" These questions serve as an important way of dealing with the unfinished business of the relationship that can potentially block successful completion of the grieving. One may feel, "How can I let her go if I never told her how much she meant to me?"

A possible hindrance to the successful completion of the process of grief therapy is the difficulty some students have with ambiguity and maturational conflicts about autonomy. This seems to affect the students' active incorporation or assimilation of the deceased. In the process of selective identification the student chooses those aspects such as traits, strengths, or guiding principles of the deceased that are worthy of incorporation into the ego ideal. Remnants of childhood's magical thinking still appear in this age group.

They seem to fear the total loss of the deceased if they let
go and stop mourning. The fear is that nothing will be left
of the relationship, that they will feel as if it had never
existed. Students usually need help in understanding that
they have already incorporated the deceased into their lives
(in other words, that the person "lives" on in them and that
they can continue to selectively incorporate further).

For certain of those students who have good ego strength,
it may be helpful occasionally to utilize gestalt techniques.
These therapeutic tools can be powerful but they need to be
used judiciously, with attention to timing, by experienced
therapists trained in the employment of such techniques.
Melges and DeMaso (1980) describe a guided imagery technique
of talking with the deceased and Tobin (1971) utilizes the
"empty chair" technique to do the same. These tools are
especially useful in helping clients who are experiencing
difficulty in saying a final goodbye.

The case of Ellie illustrates the use of this technique
and the idea of continued incorporation. Ellie was a graduate student whose father had died 16 years earlier. Her
unresolved grief and irrational guilt about his death had
led to years of self-defeating behavior. Although she had
completed most of her mourning tasks, she seemed unable to
make the final break by saying a last goodbye. Utilizing the
empty chair she was able to loudly express her anger toward
him and to state that she must let him go "because I can't
continue to let you cause me this much pain." She was able
to express regrets at what had been missing in their relationship, but also to acknowledge the positive aspects of her
father that she would continue to incorporate into her life.
"There are parts of you I will always carry with me but I
have to let you go and say goodbye now."

It is appropriate to move toward termination when client
and therapist sense that the student is returning to the pre-
loss equilibrium. Typically, after successful treatment
clients become aware of feeling quite different subjectively.
"I seem to be able to talk about her without crying now."
"I went four days without a single thought of my father! I
haven't done this since his death." Clients report more positive feelings about the deceased, too. They can focus on
positive memories they wish to retain rather than on feelings
of anger or sadness. There are behavioral changes as well.
The phrase "rejoining the living" is appropriate. Completed
grief work should result in the client's resuming normal
activities, beginning to socialize more, and investing in new
relationships. As Worden (1982) observes, "Grief therapy
works. Unlike some other psychotherapies, in which one may
not be certain about the effectiveness and efficacy of the
treatment, grief therapy can be very effective. The subjective experiences and observable behavioral changes lend cre-

dence to the value of such targeted therapetuic intervention."

It is often helpful to examine the client's usual coping
styles and defenses. The counselor needs to explore how
effective these defenses were in dealing with this particular
loss to determine how the coping style might be altered or
the defenses consolidated in order to deal more effectively
with future difficulties and losses. The student should
always be helped by means of anticipatory planning for times
when the sense of loss might be reactivated, such as holiday
seasons, anniversaries, and milestone events like college
graduation or a wedding. The student's sense of mastery is
aided by being able to purposefully plan for these events and
the feelings that may be generated. This provides a bridge
from the past to the future. Many students choose to add a
ritual or memorial to these times. For example, one student
whose mother died picked two items of her mother's jewelry to
wear, one at graduation and one at her wedding, to acknowledge the feelings she had for her mother and her desire for
the mother's presence at these landmark life events. Another
student chose to read his deceased father's favorite Christmas story aloud to the family on Christmas Eve every year as
an ongoing memorial. Around the time of her unfulfilled
delivery date after her abortion, yet a third student began
a major educational project that was her memorial to the lost
child but was also a recognition of the need to move on with
her life.

Termination of therapy is a particularly crucial phase
of grief work since it is a recapitulation of the process of
separation and loss. With the time-limited contract, however,
the termination is explicit and should be discussed throughout
the course of treatment. It may be helpful for students to
pick their actual date of termination themselves. Increasing
the interval between sessions near the end of treatment may
be used as a way of testing their abilities in confronting
issues on their own.

The therapist should encourage the student to translate
the concepts learned in treatment about the loss process to
the termination situation. "Knowing what you know now about
saying goodbye, I wonder how you could apply that to us and
our saying goodbye." Emphasis, here too, is placed on reviewing the relationship, expressing emotions and ambivalence,
and considering the "mad, glad, and sad" feelings. Students
typically handle this task with relative ease compared to the
difficulty they had with their previous loss, although some
sadness can still be expected. The termination process is
reinforcing and heightens the student's sense of mastery over
the previous loss that led to counseling. It also helps in
recognizing newly acquired skills and the ability to make the
transition to the future with its inevitable losses.

Countertransference Issues

Many therapists steer clear of grief work because of their own discomfort with grief. Bowlby (1980) states, "The loss of a loved person is one of the most intensely painful experiences any human being can suffer, and not only is it painful to experience, but also painful to witness. . . ." In grief work, as in all clinical work, there is challenge and there can be frustration, when the therapist's own feelings and resistances, as well as those of the client, are provoked. As we review another's loss, we are inescapably reminded of our own losses. Thus it may be particularly problematic if the therapist's loss is recent, unresolved, or is similar to the client's loss. Granet and Kalman (1982) point out the need for therapists not only to monitor their own losses and defenses, but also be particularly aware of their own anniversary reactions. Worden (1982) suggests that grief work may also provoke the counselor's fear of future losses as well as the client's. Finally, just as the student is challenged existentially by confronting the inevitability of death, so are we.

The counselor hoping to do grief work needs to address these issues directly by reviewing personal past losses, recalling what was helpful and what was not helpful in the grieving process and examining the degree of resolution achieved. Therapists with recent major losses may find grief work arduous and may be less effective than usual in their work. Therapists should allow themselves to refrain from assisting others in grief work until personal losses are less immediate and a sense of resolution to their mourning process is accomplished. Conversely, the therapist who has experienced and worked through a severe loss is in a unique position to empathize and to make creative therapeutic use of personal experience. The therapist can constructively use the empathy to reach into the self for examples of what loss and grief can be like. This modeling enables the student to know that the counselor is existentially able to relate to the experience and further promotes the alliance along with the client's sense of freedom to express feelings. Examples of modeling include: "Have you ever noticed that everything reminds you of the person you've lost?" and "I wonder if you've had the sensation of thinking you've seen the person who has died?"

Although difficult, because so much affect is mobilized, grief counseling offers therapists some unique opportunities such as the ability to share in a different way in clients' lives, hearing very special memories, "meeting" special people, and often dealing with less conflictual material than usual. Also, there is the sense of achievement in having helped a student over a major hurdle. While therapists

should not use clients to meet personal needs, there is no
question that we are enriched by our relationships and
experiences with them. Grief therapy provides us with the
chance to become more comfortable with loss and to be able
to tolerate better this truly universal issue.

Referral

The therapist needs to recognize the limits of short-term
therapy and begin to make preparations for referral for
longer-term therapy when an attempt at brief grief work has
been found to be unsuccessful. Clients not likely to benefit
from brief grief therapy and who thus need referral include
those with very brittle defenses, those for whom the inhibi-
tion of affect is too great to allow the necessary expression
of feeling, and those whose rage is so powerful that it
threatens to overwhelm their defenses. Personality difficulties such as these make the focused, goal-oriented treatment
inappropriate. Only after further therapy with persons experienced in long-term treatment may it be possible for these
clients to resolve their loss and grief.

It is important to help such a student see the referral
for long-term therapy outside the service as not just another
narcissistic injury to one who has already suffered a loss,
but rather to promote the view that the crisis is an opportunity to work through some issues that would otherwise cause
trouble. In this way, the premise that "every crisis is an
opportunity for growth," which underlies the brief treatment
described, holds true even for those with whom short-term work
is not enough.

REFERENCES

Barry, M.J. "The Prolonged Grief Reaction." *Mayo Clinic
Proceedings* 48 (1973):329-335.

---. "Therapeutic Experience With Patients Referred for
Prolonged Grief Reaction--Some Second Thoughts." *Mayo
Clinic Proceedings* 56 (1981):744-748.

Bowlby, J. "Processes of Mourning." *International Journal
of Psychoanalysis* 42 (July-October 1961):317-340.

---. "Attachment and Loss." In *Loss, Sadness, and Depression.* New York: Basic Books, 1980.

Chickering, A.W. *Education and Identity.* San Francisco:
Jossey-Bass, 1972.

Clayton, P., L. Desmarais, and G. Winokur. "A Study of Normal Bereavement." *American Journal of Psychiatry* 125 (1968):168-170.

Engel, G.L. "A Group Dynamic Approach to Teaching and Learning about Grief." *Omega: Journal of Death and Dying* 12 (1981):1-13.

Farnsworth, D.L. *Psychiatry, Education, and the Young Adult.* Springfield, Ill.: Thomas, 1966.

Granet, R.B. and T.P. Kalman. "Anniversary Reactions in Therapists." *American Journal of Psychiatry* 139 (1982): 1599-1600.

Kushner, S. *When Bad Things Happen to Good People.* New York: Schocken Books, 1981.

LaGrand, L.E. "Loss Reactions of College Students: A Descriptive Analysis." *Death Education* 5 (1981):235-248.

Lindemann, E. "Symptomatology and Management of Acute Grief." *American Journal of Psychiatry* 101 (1944):141.

Margolin, C. "Evaluating Suicide Potential in the Emergency Department." *Journal of Emergency Nursing* 3 (1977):21-25.

Melges, F.T. and D.R. DeMaso. "Grief Resolution Therapy: Reliving, Revising, and Revisiting." *American Journal of Psychotherapy* 34 (1980):51-61.

Parkes, C.M. *Bereavement: A Study of Grief in Adult Life.* London: Tavistock, 1972.

Rapoport, L. "The State of Crisis: Some Theoretical Considerations. In *Crisis Intervention: Selected Readings*, edited by H. Parad. New York: Family Service Association, 1965. Pp. 5-21.

Rees, W.D. "The Bereaved and Their Hallucinations." In *Bereavement: Its Psychosocial Aspects*, edited by B. Schoenberg. New York: Columbia University Press, 1975.

Sustento, J.D. "Acute Grief Reaction." In *Handbook of Psychiatry*, edited by P. Solomon and V. Patch. Canada: Lange Medical Publications, 1969.

Tobin, S.A. "Saying Goodbye in Gestalt Therapy." *Psychotherapy: Theory, Research, and Practice* 8 (1971):150-155.

Werner, A. and M.D. Jones. "Parent Loss in College Students." *Journal of the American College Health Association* 27 (1979):253-256.

Worden, J.W. *Grief Counseling and Grief Therapy: A Handbook for the Mental Health Practitioner.* New York: Springer, 1982.

5

Psychodynamic Issues in Vocational Counseling

Joseph E. Talley

The purpose of vocational counseling as described here is to enable the student to select a tentative vocational direction with an awareness of sufficient information about the "world of work" as well as relevant information about "the self." The former refers to considerations of salary, supply and demand factors in the job market, entry level requirements for certain occupations, and what the day to day activities are in occupations of interest to the student. Self information includes the student's skills and abilities, interests, values, and salient personality traits. Acknowledging that the only way to be sure one feels satisfied in an occupation is to try it, the vocational direction decision is described as tentative, underscoring the fact that it is alterable and subject to change.

The actual process of vocational counseling as it has most often been done consists of first establishing a comfortable working relationship with the student, then assessing together the information needed and obtaining it. Finally, the decision-making process is engaged in leading to the conclusion of counseling. Decision-making concerns might include how much weight to give the different factors under consideration, conflicts with parents or others about the choice, and significant internal conflicts about the options. It is critical to ascertain how the student thinks the best choice will be recognized. Will it just feel right? Will all doubts cease? Will others all find it a good decision?

Although traditionally vocational counseling would work with decision-making strategies if necessary, it appears that a crucial question is overlooked in this process. Specifically, how does it come to be that this particular student seeks vocational counseling and others do not? This question is especially pertinent for those students who seem unable to

benefit from the process as described. Typically, we conclude that the student wisely seeks counseling to get valuable preparation for the future, or we focus on the rationale
that selecting a vocation is a normal developmental task with
which the student understandably wants help. While both of
these reasons are true for many students, there are certainly
numbers of students for whom this is not the case. This is
made apparent by the fact that students often do not seek
readily available information that would be helpful to the
counseling process, as well as by the observation that many
appear unable to make even a tentative decision despite ample
information and the assistance of decision-making strategies.
At this juncture it is difficult to avoid the conclusion that
for these students there is some obstruction to choosing a
vocation other than the lack of ingredients provided in
traditional vocational counseling. It appears that such persons for some reason need, at least at this time, to avoid
selecting a direction.

Many obstacles involving "readiness" to choose may sub-
side with time alone. However, if readiness is affected by
personality factors some attention to these factors should
enhance the counseling process. Thus, personality traits or
psychodynamic issues may become part of the domain of vocational counseling. This poses a problem since the student
coming for vocational counseling usually does not expect to
explore personality variables inhibiting vocational choice.
Proceeding with such an exploration hastily or without a
sufficiently mutual collaborative effort may result in the
student feeling intruded upon and pushed into a therapy situation. Therefore, a gentle transition with which the student
feels comfortable is essential. One means of doing this is
to note the importance of occupational fit to personality and
then proceed with asking how the student sees his or her
personality including the very useful aspects, as well as the
traits that might be constricting or limiting. An exploration of this type gives some feel for how comfortable the
student is with self evaluation and how capable the student
is at self observation.

In essence, most people coming for vocational counseling
are saying, "Look there's really nothing wrong with me but I
need help in choosing a career." They want to see the problem as situational and indeed it may be. However, for those
students not benefitted by a "developmental/situational"
approach, the counselor needs to get around to saying in so
many words, "Yes, right. There's really nothing 'wrong' with
you, but might there be something important about how you're
going about this task that is making it more difficult, and
if we could together find out what it is we'd be a step further down the road?" Such a transition might be done after
the general personality considerations regarding occupations
have been discussed.

The approach put forth here is for use with a certain group of students seeking vocational counseling. For many the traditional approach described is sufficient; for others there are personality problems so profound that psychotherapy will be necessary before functioning in the world of work is possible. For yet a third group traditional vocational counseling will be helpful but not sufficient to overcome the internal obstacles to making a career choice. This group of students may come to make greater use of vocational counseling when it includes some work on these internal obstacles. This approach is strategic, primarily cognitive, and quite issue-focused with the aim of getting the student over the "developmental hump" in order to experience something new, in the hope that strengths will develop that can then be built on. At the theoretical level this model is similar to Milton Erickson's strategic psychotherapy that often focuses on a developmental problem. Thus, there is no direct aim toward significant personality alteration although the personality style may need brief exploration at the cognitive-behavioral level. However, this experience may over time lead to broader personality alterations.

Important technique-related phases in vocational counseling of this type include the necessity of establishing a comfortable working relationship followed by a task phase of completing as many of the traditional vocational counseling activities as possible. However, when an impasse or stalemate is reached, the focus in this model is on assisting the student in puzzling about the internal conflicts and cognitive patterns blocking progress. Work is aimed toward the goal of decreasing the intensity of the pattern so that the process of vocational choice will proceed more easily. This may be done in a collaborative and direct manner if the student wishes, but most often an indirect approach is required due to the student's lack of readiness to accept the idea that a personality problem exists. The indirect approach rests on strategically placed casual comments that speak to the student's problem without ever requiring an acknowledgement of the problem.

At each phase the approach will vary with the type of student. The entire process may occur in one session or in several and thus the phases may last from a few minutes to a few hours each. The initial phase of establishing a comfortable working relationship may begin with asking the student, "Where's a good place for us to start today?" or "What brings you to talk with me today?" Any such statement will suffice if it gives the student an opportunity to say almost anything, due to the counselor's presuming little or nothing. This leaves it up to the student to identify the focus as vocational and allows the student the option of giving one reason for coming to a professor, dean, parent, or even the receptionist at the counseling center, and then to tell the counselor that the problem is of a more personal nature. These open-ended introductions aid in assessing the student, as the response reveals how a small ambiguous task is approached and how much responsibility is assumed. This opening question also looks for what the student sees as the goal of counseling or what is hoped for from counseling.

As the process of vocational counseling commences, a number of important psychodynamic issues come into play. First, how does the student's behavior affect the relationship with the counselor? Second, how do the counselor's theoretical views and model of vocational counseling affect the relationship with the student? As the work together proceeds, the counselor might observe the student's ability to utilize the counseling process and note in which ways this student's personality traits appear to make selecting a career pathway difficult. The counselor must continue to evaluate whether these traits appear significant enough to warrant an eventual discussion of them. If so, then the method of doing this must be formulated.

In answering these questions a host of other more specific considerations are helpful, such as the following:

How passive or nonverbal is the student?

Is the student clear about what s/he wants?

What and how much is expected of the counselor?

How are these expectations communicated?

Is the student concerned with making "the right" decision?

Is changing occupations viewed as having "wasted time?"

Can the idea of compromise be tolerated or must the choice be perfect and totally satisfying?

How afraid is the student of not having all options open?

What rank or status does the student appear to assign the counselor?

Does the student relate as if the counselor were a servant, all-knowing professional, or another person with something valuable to offer?

The answers to these questions are particularly useful in ascertaining whether the student is adequately described by one of three personality-style categories. Although there may be other personality traits and styles that obstruct vocational counseling, I have found the ones that appear most

frequently are the following: (1) the passive-dependent
student; (2) the student with self-esteem or narcissistic
problems; and (3) the obsessive-perfectionistic student.
Asking the student what specifically is appealing or unap-
pealing about any occupations currently under consideration
gives a sense of what motivates the student and what is
important for the student to avoid. Pieced together this
information might suggest, for example, that being publicly
recognized is highly desired and being unnoticed, feared.
Such information is helpful as problem-solving data, too,
since it brings the focus to the particulars of a vocation.
Questions might be posed by the counselor to glean more
material of this nature such as "What would it be like for
you to be . . ." (for example, a lawyer in a large prestigious firm doing legal research)? It may be discovered that
doing research does not permit sufficient interaction with
people, or that being on the bottom of the group hierarchy
is more of a cost than being in a presitgious firm is a
benefit. All of this information reveals the nature of the
student's values and personality preferences. Having the
student react to questions such as, "How would you feel
about being a ---?" can make the student's relevant wishes
and fears evident.

THE PASSIVE-DEPENDENT STUDENT

    The passive-dependent style student demonstrates an
expectation that all relevant information will be provided
with little or no effort on the student's part. Easily
accessible written materials will be ignored in favor of
asking the professional for all the facts. Thus the counselor is set up as all-knowing and therefore capable of meeting
the student's needs to be dependent. Such behavior reveals
a wish to be taken care of by someone who is perceived as
both powerful and nurturing. When asked questions for reflection, these students frequently give the rebuttal, "I
don't know." If questions are posed about the "I don't know"
responses, the student may resort to saying, "Well, that's
what I came here to find out." When the counselor does not
gratify the passive-dependent client's wish to be told what
to do, the expectations may shift to psychometric instruments
such as interest inventories. The basic attempt of the
passive-dependent student is to get someone or something else
to be responsible for the decision since the student feels
unable to assume a task of such magnitude. In some part of
the student's mind, accepting this responsibility would be
an admission that there is no strong, protective caretaker
and therefore making a decision feels, at least for the
moment, like a loss because it frustrates the wish to remain

in a childlike mode. Of course, there may be other complications regarding the use of passivity as a manipulative
means or passivity as an expression of anger. Nevertheless,
there is the loss of whatever benefits have been gained
from this interpersonal posture if change occurs. Specifics
of this naturally vary from person to person.

The passive-dependent student may begin with a series of
ambiguous replies immediately from the outset, when asked
what is wanted from counseling, such as, "Well, I'm really
not sure." The response, "For you to tell me what I should
do," has been heard more than once. Although the obsessive
student may also reply with "I'm not really sure," subsequent questions about interests and previous vocational
thoughts will yield more than a repetition of, "I don't know"
and "That's what I came here to find out" statements, typical
of overly passive students. A productive working relationship is often impossible to establish with extremely passive-
dependent individuals because of his or her expectation that
the counselor will provide all and ask for little participation. If a collaborative effort cannot be established, then
the counselor may choose between puzzling with the student
about the evident difficulty in reflecting on the questions
posed, and pointing out the great limitations of the counseling process if the student is not actively engaged. Benign
clarification regarding what the counselor can and cannot
provide is often helpful in this situation. However, clarification of this sort may be perceived as critical if not
timed well and done gently. A poor handling of this may push
the student into an even more passive stance or prompt the
termination of counseling.

Another option is to gratify some of the dependency
wishes by offering possibilities such as interest inventories, values clarification inventories, and relevant personality assessment tools in order to convey a willingness to
actively help and be concerned about the student. This
avenue gives more time for a working relationship to develop
and increases the likelihood of a less threatened response
if it appears necessary to discuss the student's difficulty
in actively participating. This group of students is in all
probability the easiest to alienate and for some students no
amount of nurturance will seem sufficient and no means of
addressing the issue will prove productive. An approach
beginning with nurturance through information or test results,
coupled with overt praise for whatever active responses are
made, should provide the best background for a nonauthoritar-
ian and cautious focus on the passivity. This may be initiated by asking the student about expectations of how counseling would proceed, meaning what the counselor would do and
what the student would contribute. Some orientation regarding how the process might best work may be done or repeated

at this time. In a more direct discussion of how the student is responding, it is very possible that the counselor will be perceived as critical or blaming. This is often obviated by framing the matter as a clarification of the process and what the student can do to most benefit from "working together." The back and forth of passivity and clarification may recur throughout the tasks of vocational counseling and appear again in its most intense form with dependent features at the decision-making phase. At this time a focus on how it feels for the student to assume such responsibility coupled with encouragement from the counselor is usually the best strategy for continuing momentum through the tentative choice phase. Thus the personality dynamics may need to be addressed directly or indirectly with the passive-dependent student quite early in the work and usually examined more than once at impasses during counseling.

THE STUDENT WITH SELF-ESTEEM OR
NARCISSISTIC PROBLEMS

The student with variable self-esteem or narcissistic concerns shows a second personality trait that can become entangled with vocational choice. These students attempt to salvage self-esteem by choosing a prestigious vocation. This may be seen as an effort to compensate for a lack of self-esteem in other areas of life or as an attempt to insulate a fragile sense of self from assault on self-esteem. Consequently, actualizing the prestigious vocational choice comes to feel like a matter of life and death for the sense of self-worth. It is common for the student with narcissistic concerns to wish to start at the top of a profession without going through the arduous process of working upward over time. For example, a student may want to become a judge without the "drudgery" of law school or "the mundaneness" of being an attorney. Another student may wish to be a professor and plan to attend graduate school as a means to this end with no substantive interest in the subject matter itself. Such individuals long for respect and admiration and see a prestigious occupation as the necessary means to obtain it. While some measure of this is true for many students, those with severe self-esteem issues are inclined to believe that being a member of a certain profession will place them beyond criticism and compel deference regardless of their other behavior. One student with self-esteem issues constantly feared being "one of the nameless and the faceless" and becoming a famous physicist was to be his guarantee against this. It is noteworthy how he looked with disdain upon most other people and did not see them as significant (to illustrate, "He is not a force to be reckoned with"). Another student with narcissistic concerns felt that he must (and was destined to) become a great writer. He once likened himself to Vincent Van Gogh in a song lyric that went, "But I could have told you Vincent, this world was never meant for one as beautiful as you." The student seemed concerned that the counselor pay continued intense attention to him, but related in such a way as to indicate that he did not see the counselor as a person with feelings and interests in his own right. The student looking for a vocational solution to self-esteem deficits wants to be sure that the career will offer an un-limited supply of respect and admiration. Narcissistic and self-esteem concerns often appear as significant features in students whose primary personality style is most similar to one of the other two categories.

During the first encounter, the student with prominent self-esteem concerns often will manifest a muted form of what the narcissistic patient initially shows to the psychothera-pist. Therefore, the vocational counselor may be treated with some deference and be seen as having the answer to the student's problems, when the student is feeling a lack of positive self-regard. Conversely, the counselor may be per-ceived as having little skill or value and in the extreme case be perceived as a servant of sorts, when the student is feeling an inflated sense of self-regard. The working rela-tionship the student hopes for is one of "you work for me" in either case. The opening sentences and demeanor of the stu-dent often reveal such conflicts. When the student is feel-ing vulnerable and has less positive self-regard the counse-lor may be idealized, so that the student may then feel associated with a powerful ally with whom he can identify. Consequently, this type of student may seem at first appear-ance to be passive-dependent. However, a swing will eventu-ally occur to the more grandiose or inflated self as soon as a boost in self-esteem occurs, and then the attitude of superiority becomes clear. The variation in intensity of these dynamics determines the degree to which the student will demean or idealize the tasks and tools of vocational counseling as well as the counselor.

The decision-making phase with these students often focuses on the discrepancy between what is wished for and what is actually possible. This process can be particularly painful if a long-held, specific occupational dream designed to insure self-esteem seems impossible to actualize. Such a loss would result in an injury to self-esteem for most, but it is more devastating for these students to the degree that the choice was motivated by needs to preserve the sense of self through winning admiration by means of an occupation. At first no other options may be entertained as acceptable; however, with time and a supportive focus on the fact that most of the sense of loss stems from a highly idealized fantasy of how things would have been rather than a picture of what such a life style would have most likely been in reality, changes may begin.

Students with some of these mild to moderate narcissistic features are generally open to discussing how "self-image" might be associated with vocational choice and to puzzle about how realistic certain aspects of their wishes are. Nevertheless, modifications are difficult. The bulk of what can be done, until the student feels ready to ponder new options, is to begin to consider that although the vocational dream may not become reality, the student can still be a worthwhile person and enjoy life.

THE OBSESSIVE-PERFECTIONISTIC STUDENT

A third and perhaps the most frequently seen pattern is that of the obsessive, perfectionistic student. Statements these students often make include, "I want to be sure that I make the 'right' choice," "I want to be sure that I don't waste any time" and their replies are saturated with, "Yes . . ., but . . ." whenever the decision-making process is begun. The obsessive looks continually for more and more information and seems to want a guarantee that the choice will seem right forever, as if an insurance policy on the future were possible. It is particularly frustrating to these students to realize that there really is no way to know absolutely what career they will be satisfied with other than by trying it. Being perfectionistic, the word "compromise" elicits disgust and fears of becoming "mediocre." Compromising is viewed as selling out, even when the composite of what is wished for vocationally does not appear to exist. This reaction to "mediocrity" is primarily related to the fear of not *doing* one's best whereas the narcissistic student's fear of mediocrity is primarily focused on not *appearing* one's best. The obsessive's most difficult situation occurs when there are two occupations equally favored but very different in type, such as a free-lance fiction writer and a computer systems analyst. In such situations the obsessive may fear that a decision will result in the loss of a part of the self or a loss of control that was felt when both options were open. This dilemma can result in a double approach/avoidance conflict or a stalemate when all the tasks of vocational counseling have been completed except for selecting a tentative choice. It is the obsessive's perfectionistic insistence on the choice being "the right" one (guaranteed permanent satisfaction, with no compromises) that makes the decision impossible.

The vocationally obsessive, perfectionistic student is certainly made more anxious by a tight economy and an increasingly competitive job market. However, for most students the pattern is primarily supported by the parental injunction, "You are lovable only if you work extremely hard and accomplish a great deal," that has been given to many during childhood. Thus, upon approaching adulthood, when the student sees that achieving all that was hoped for is unlikely, choosing a pathway seems impossible due to the exaggerated sense of loss that is felt with a decision. No matter what variations on the theme lie under the obsessiveness and perfectionism, there are fears to be reckoned with that are being defended against by avoidance and rumination. Decreasing the fears (the avoidance gradient) enough to permit a tentative choice is the goal.

Establishing a fruitful working relationship with the obsessive student often requires some interventions to decrease anxiety before the student can work collaboratively, since the intense anxiety may leave the student internally focused to the extreme. Comments directed toward lessening the student's sense of urgency are generally helpful. It is efficacious, when possible, to show that there is actually more time to choose than the student now believes, underscoring that the time when a tentative choice must be made regarding career plans is self-imposed and arbitrary. Of course parents or deans may be colluding with these feelings of urgency, but, in fact, all choices are open to subsequent revision. Helping the student to feel less alone in this situation (universalizing) is also effective in anxiety reduction. This can be done by giving information that emphasizes that many students are experiencing the same feelings at this time. Noting the facts that most persons do not find the career from which they will retire until about 35 years of age and that, on the average, Americans engage in three different careers in a lifetime demonstrates that at some time everyone has experienced similar conflicts. Relaxation or imagery exercises may lessen anxiety for those obsessives who feel comfortable doing them. For other anxious students listening to their interests or allowing the ventilation of concerns will lead to increased comfort internally and subsequently to more comfort with the counselor. Focusing on relaxation as a task the student must "try to work on" is counterproductive. It should be framed as something to be allowed to happen with little or no effort. A brief but focused series of psychotherapeutic interventions to decrease anxiety about change and loosen cognitive rigidity through imagery or sensate focusing exercises (Lazarus 1976) has proven effective.

Once some degree of relaxation has been achieved, listening to the student's vocational thoughts to date should build the rapport. Most importantly, challenging rigid, perfectionistic thinking should be avoided at this time as should

any control struggles. Allowing the student to select what
appears most helpful from what the counselor can offer gives
the message that the student's individuality and judgment is
respected.

When a comfortable working relationship has been established, the tasks of vocational counseling may be set up in
such a way as to best work with the obsessive by attempting
to amplify feelings associated with different vocations.
Helping the obsessive visualize (with eyes closed if this can
be done comfortably) what a specific vocation may be like
often taps relevant feelings. On the other hand, interest
inventories and other psychometric approaches appeal to this
type of student's desire for structure. Some balance between
the familiar and the new in the approach provides both comfort and challenge for the student.

Moving into the decision-making phase, the student may
become increasingly obsessive and continually feel the need
for more and more information. In the deliberations and
ruminations the counselor may be helpful by periodically
inquiring about what the student would find enjoyable in a
specific occupation. This shifts the focus from the cognitive to the effective dimension often ignored by the obsessive. The perfectionistic trait makes giving up one thing
in order to gain something else difficult and as it becomes
evident that the student seems unable to accept a compromise
with its inherent loss and gain balance, turning the focus
to the internal difficulty may be timely. A sensitive,
gradual but straightforward look at the student's insistence
on holding out for all that is wished for and for some form
of guarantee that the choice will be found right throughout
life should always be posed in a manner that allows the student to reject the idea if it is too distressing at the
present time. Nevertheless such a realistic presentation
may result in the student's acceptance that knowing what the
future holds is impossible. From this point a tentative
choice may be made with the notion that, "Yes, something is
lost in making a choice but there are much greater losses if
a choice is not made."

It has been my experience that the obsessive, perfectionistic student is the most likely of the three types to engage
in a less defensive discussion of the personality trait. In
order to demonstrate to the student that the thinking style
is the primary issue and not the particular situation, sup-
porting data may be gleaned from looking at the student's
decision-making history for romantic commitments, large pur-
chases, or significant time commitments. During decision
making, the clear identification of the gains and losses
associated with each vocational choice under consideration
aids in keeping a concrete focus. Although it is not the
focus of this discussion, it is possible that a career choice

not yet considered exists that will enhance gains and minimize losses. Despite the fact that the student may be hoping
for a completely ideal solution, the counselor should not
advocate the abandonment of the search for a satisfying fit
until all knowable possibilities have been considered.

To summarize, each of the three personality styles
examined bring different psychodynamic themes into the work.
Yet there is a commonality in that the difficulty in making
progress centers around the wish for something and the fear
of loss. The passive-dependent student wishes to be nur-
tured and fears personal responsibility because it represents
the loss of being taken care of and protected. The student
with self-esteem problems wishes to be admired and for his or
her self-worth to be beyond question. The fear is that shame
and humiliation will occur if the vocation is not prestigious
enough to defend against any doubts or assaults to self-worth.
For the obsessive student there is a wish to have control over
the future by selecting the perfectly satisfying choice and
yet a fear that making such a choice will result in the loss
of the control found in "keeping all options open," as well
as the losses that will result from any compromises. Thus,
staying at an impasse as to vocational decision can be a
defense against loss for all three of these groups. However,
the nature of the loss is different for each and consequently
technique and focus will vary depending on the nature of the
loss and other variables relevant to the particular individual. Finally, a combination of these personality traits is
common and many students with the initial appearance of an
obsessive may have significant self-esteem issues regarding
career choice. In such cases, both issues must be identified
and worked with in order for the student to benefit.

In conclusion, it is interesting to note how rarely professionals in vocational counseling seem to consider psychodynamic issues as relevant in their work. There appears to
be a bias toward accepting the presenting problem as is, with
little if any attention given to the possibility that such
presentations are not necessarily "developmental" problems
alone. Mastering a developmental task is certainly more difficult for those with problematic personality traits and this
population does not receive adequate help unless both the
developmental problems and the intrapsychic dilemmas are
dealt with. The most important key in the judicious use of
such a combined approach is ascertaining if and when the
student is ready to consider personality traits as important.
If it is felt that the suggestion to consider personality
traits as important material would be experienced by the student as intrusive or if the psychodynamic issues appear
severe enough to warrant long-term psychotherapy, then the
direct aspects of this approach should not be employed and
the indirect methods should be used cautiously, if at all.

REFERENCES

Erickson, Milton H., Ernest L. Rossi, and Sheila I. Rossi.
    Hypnotic Realities. New York: Irvington, 1976.

Lazarus, A.A. *Multimodal Behavior Therapy*. New York:
    Springer, 1976.

6

Perfectionistic Thinking in University Students: Implications for Individual Treatment

Carol A. Moore and John C. Barrow

INTRODUCTION

Sara was a 19-year-old sophomore enrolled in a medium-sized state university. She was referred to the student mental health center by her academic advisor as a result of her repeated inability to complete and hand in her English composition assignments. Sara reported her initial concern in coming to the mental health center as being an inability to complete her assignments due to escalating depression and fears that she would be given an "F." She described having received a "C" on her first practice paper in English and stated that she had not completed an assignment since then. She described episodes of crying when she tried to write, "drawing a blank," and pervasive feelings of failure and worthlessness. Sara reported being the oldest of three children from an upper-middle-class family in which her father was a lawyer and her mother a housewife with a bachelor's degree in education. Sara had been unable to tell her parents of her difficulties because she feared they would be disappointed. She stated that she had made "all As" in high school, had written for the school newspaper, and had always enjoyed writing in the past.

Sara is similar to many students referred to university student mental health and counseling centers. Although her reported symptoms resemble those which accompany a variety of diagnosable situational-emotional disturbances including mild depression and obsessive-compulsive disorder, they are largely contained within the category of "nondiagnosable disorders" and, as such, may prove difficult to assess and treat effectively. The absence of appropriate classifications for these nondiagnosable disorders coupled with the prevalence of these kinds of concerns in a university population suggest that student mental health service providers must begin to consider assessment and intervention ideas different from those that have traditionally been considered useful. Cognitive assessment is one such novel intervention approach that has been found to be effective in the assessment and treatment of these kinds of problems (Burns 1980a; Ellis & Harper 1975; Meichenbaum 1977). The cognitive approach involves identifying a specific cognitive style that may underlie symptoms, and targeting that style as a possible area for intervention.

A re-examination of the case of Sara from a cognitive perspective reveals a thread of continuity between her initial concerns and the dynamics of her case as depicted in her perfectionistic cognitive style. This perfectionistic thinking, which is consistent with her academic and familial history, may be integrally related to her depression, writing block, procrastination, and academic difficulty.

The purpose of this chapter is to discuss the use of cognitive assessment and intervention with perfectionistic thinking in university students. The discussion will include the distinctions between perfectionistic cognitive style and related "diagnoses," an exploration of the development of perfectionistic thinking in college students, and, finally, implications for the individual treatment of students who are restricted by their perfectionistic cognitive styles.

THE PERFECTIONISTIC COGNITIVE STYLE

Defining Perfectionistic Thinking

A definition of perfectionistic thinking and a discussion of its elements have been offered by Barrow and Moore (1983) and Burns (1980b). Reiterated here, perfectionistic cognitive style, also referred to as perfectionistic thinking, can be defined as a network of cognitions, including expectations, interpretations of events, and evaluations of oneself and others, characterized by (1) the setting of unrealistic standards and expectations, (2) rigid, unrelenting, and indiscriminate adherence to these standards, and (3) the equating of self-worth with performance. Common elements of perfectionistic thinking include the following:

1. Dichotomous, "all-or-none" thinking is frequent. Experiences and self tend to be viewed in polarities, such as success-failure or saint-sinner.
2. Goals are rigidified and seen as necessities for self-esteem rather than as standards to use in motivating one's behavior. "I want" becomes "I need" or "I must" in the person's mind.

3. Similarly, desires are transformed into demands, and "I would like" becomes "I should-must-ought to have."

4. Time perception is affected, in that in perfectionistic thinking a student is often excessively future-focused. This phenomenon can be thought of as the "hurdle effect," in that the student's attention is so focused upon the hurdles ahead that there is little appreciation of the hurdles already cleared.

5. "Telescoping," another distortion of time perception, occurs when unmet goals or demands are initially magnified out of proportion. When a goal is met, however, it is as though the student looks through the telescope in reverse and the met goals are suddenly viewed as relatively unimportant.

6. In this process, selective attention acts as a perfectionistic filter, such that attained goals become devalued or ignored, while unattained goals are magnified and flaws scrutinized. The net effect is that it is very difficult to win and easy to lose.

7. As a result of the above thinking patterns, very little self-reward is given for accomplishments. There is little time devoted to savoring a success or positive experience.

8. Being "average" or "ordinary" in an important activity comes to be seen as shameful. The dichotomous thinking previously mentioned is activated and the student views him/herself as either superlative or a failure.

9. A compulsive cycle is often established and an addictive adherence to perfectionistic thinking is maintained. Perfectionistic standards produce debilitating emotions such as anxiety and frustration that may actually interfere with and limit performance. When performance is unacceptable, the student resolves to try harder and "be perfect" the next time, thus perpetuating the cycle.

The Role of Perfectionistic Thinking

The role of perfectionistic thinking can be best understood by using Ellis's cognitive analysis system (Ellis & Harper 1975). At point A, the antecedent event, a student's perfectionistic tendencies are triggered by a certain situation, for instance a deadline, or test, or a social event. If the student responds at point B, the belief about the antecedent event, with a perfectionistic belief or way of thinking and interpreting the situation, various affective and behavioral consequences are likely to occur at point C (the consequence), including anxiety, depression, guilt, procrastination, and compulsive behavior. If these consequences are debilitating or unwanted they may limit rather than enhance the student's performance and subsequently the student may seek help at the student mental health center, as did Sara.

Distinctions

Perfectionistic thinking can be distinguished from similar syndromes. It differs from "perfectionism" in that perfectionistic thinking implies a cognitive pattern that many people employ at different times to varying degrees and thus can be changed; "perfectionism" implies a trait that one does or does not possess and therefore may be relatively unchangeable.

Perfectionistic thinking is distinguished from "obsessive style" and "compulsive personality disorder," as classified in the DSM III, in that it is less expansive. While perfectionistic cognitive style may be one of five characteristics possessed by an individual diagnosed as a compulsive personality type, it is not the only one. Others include the restricted ability to express warmth, indecisiveness, excessive devotion to work at the expense of interpersonal relationships, and insistence that others submit to the compulsive's way of doing things (American Psychiatric Association 1981).

Perfectionistic thinking may also be inappropriately confused with overachievement and/or Type A personality. It should be noted that overachievement may be one possible behavioral pattern or response to perfectionistic thinking. Other responses include procrastination, writing blocks, depression, and hence, underachievement. Likewise, Type A personalities, as defined by Friedman and Rosenman (1974), may exhibit perfectionistic thinking; however, students with perfectionistic cognitive styles do not necessarily conform to all aspects of the Type A personality. For example, the underlying hostility and open competition of Type A persons may not be apparent in the college student with a perfectionistic cognitive style.

THE DEVELOPMENT OF PERFECTIONISTIC THINKING

In order for counselors and mental health service providers to effectively assess and treat students, some understanding of the development of this restrictive perfectionistic cognitive style in college students can be helpful. Unfortunately, no definitive experimental research is available in the area. However, from our clinical experiences and review of relevant literature, we have constructed a tentative model that has helped guide our work and made sense to students. It is likely that perfectionistic thinking is largely a result of early environmental influence. Alfred Adler proposed that birth order and family atmosphere may influence an individual to "strive for superiority," to overcome inferiorities. According to Adler, this striving may lead the individual to make possible "basic mistakes" and

cognitive distortions, such as selective perception and over-
generalization, characteristic of those made by students with
perfectionistic cognitive styles (Ansbacher & Ansbacher 1956).
Rogers (1951) has suggested that in some instances of early
development, a child may learn "conditions of worth" wherein
the child believes that regard from significant others is
conditional upon performance. If, as Rogers purports, self-
regard is an internalization of the regard extended by important others, it follows that self-worth may be seen to be
dependent upon performance, a belief that is at the core of
the perfectionistic cognitive style.

Several familial scenarios can be identified that may
lead to the fusing of self-worth with performance in the
perfectionistic thinker. If one or both parents are unduly
critical of the child and only mistakes are attended to in
the family, the child may come to believe that perfect behavior is the only way of avoiding aversive interactions. Conversely, if a child receives excessive praise and attention
for special talents and is rewarded for high grades and success anticipated for the future, that child may come to infer
that less-than perfect behavior is worthless, unacceptable,
and degrading. Inconsistent or nonexistent feedback can also
result in a child learning perfectionistic cognitions. In
the absence of external standards, the child may fill the
vacuum by setting perfection as the standard (Hamachek 1978).
Finally, perfectionistic thinking and behavior can result
from observational learning: A child may use as a model an
overly perfectionistic adult and may unknowingly introject
patterns of perfectionistic behavior and thought.

Once established, the tendency toward perfectionistic
thinking may be maintained by a variety of factors, especially the already active cognitive distortions and selective
perception indicative of perfectionistic thought. Success
experiences may be attributed to the perfectionistic beliefs
and strivings, while negative feedback is experienced as a
sign of self-inadequacy rather than as an indicator that the
basic perfectionistic assumptions are maladaptive. The intermittent reinforcement or pay-off for the perfectionistic
style serves to maintain it, in that the response pattern
established by a variable ratio schedule of reinforcement is
more difficult to extinguish than one conditioned by a continuous schedule (Burns 1980b).

Further, the heroes of commercials, movies, and television, who outwardly appear to be perfect, provide unrealistic
models thus perpetuating the perfectionistic thought process
already active in a child's mind. Finally, the emphasis
within the educational system on achievement and perfection
may maintain and further the development of perfectionistic
thinking.

We believe that adoption of a perfectionistic cognitive
style, therefore, appears to begin in early childhood and may

be maintained or exacerbated by various familial and cultural factors. The deleterious consequences of perfectionistic thinking may not actually be recognized until the period of late adolescence or young adulthood when a student has entered college and is facing an increased workload and more difficult courses than previously encountered. At this point, the student may find the perfectionistic expectations and aspirations unattainable and burdensome, and this in turn often results in depression, procrastination, or other problems. The various developmental issues encountered by the student during this stage of life, including the establishment of autonomy and identity (Chickering 1969), and the differentiation of values and expectations from those assimilated from parents, as well as the environmental demands, such as the escalating challenges of school, work, and different interpersonal relationships may combine to make the previously effective perfectionistic cognitive patterns no longer as effective for the student (Burns 1980b). Therefore, a "period of permeability" may occur in which the student is open to questioning and restructuring the perfectionistic cognitive system.

Student mental health counselors and clinicians often see the casualties that result from the ineffectiveness of the perfectionistic style, such as in the case of Sara. A familiarity with this proposed model of development of perfectionistic thinking may facilitate the appropriate assessment of students who are hampered by debilitating perfectionistic cognitive patterns. Counselors and therapists can then use the period of permeability as an opportunity for intervention and restructuring of destructive perfectionistic cognitions for the toubled student.

INDIVIDUAL INTERVENTION STRATEGIES

A variety of intervention strategies for treating students with self-defeating perfectionistic cognitive styles may be identified. The model of development discussed provides a rich framework for the general premise underlying our individualized intervention strategies: If the pattern is largely learned, the interventions must include the unlearning of destructive perfectionistic cognitive patterns and the relearning of a productive cognitive style through such techniques as modeling, feedback, practice, and the enhancement of cognitive coping skills. Interventions may be designed and implemented through either an individual or a group format. Readers interested in designing group interventions may find a previously written article helpful (Barrow & Moore 1983). Our goal in this chapter is to describe how the model applies to a short-term individual psychotherapy intervention.

Goals and General Orientation

The individual interventions we recommend for treating the perfectionistic college student have the same goals as do our group interventions: (1) to help the student become more discriminating in setting standards and goals, (2) to help the the student develop more tolerance for the inevitable times when goals are not met, (3) to help in beginning to differentiate self-worth from performance, and (4) to help develop a cognitive coping process that enables moderation and control of initial perfectionistic responses. Our interventions are designed to facilitate developmental progression and to increase awareness of suitable alternatives to ineffective perfectionistic thinking. Our aim therefore is to provide preventive intervention as well as remediation.

The interventions we suggest provide a structured format in keeping with the current emphasis upon short-term time-limited approaches (Mann 1973; Malan 1976); however, it is our hope to stimulate exploration and experimentation that will be useful to a variety of practitioners within their own individual styles. We encourage the incorporation of the ideas presented here within other ongoing intervention techniques.

Our intervention model consists of four phases: assessment, developing self-awareness, restructuring perfectionistic thinking, and termination.

Phase I: Assessment

An initial phase of assessment is crucial for effectively intervening with an individual student presenting a self-defeating perfectionistic cognitive style. During this phase a thorough exploration of the presenting concern reported by the student is undertaken and the history of the problem is explored to determine if perfectionistic thinking is indeed the appropriate target for intervention. In keeping with our ideas concerning the development of perfectionistic thinking, it is helpful to examine academic and family history including birth order, parent's expectations of the student, the accomplishments of siblings and peer group influences in order to uncover the developmental pattern of perfectionistic thinking and the factors that may be maintaining it. This history taking is beneficial for several reasons. Specifically, it allows the counselor to begin to identify perfectionistic "self-talk," a manifestation of the perfectionistic style. These self-statements will later be an important target for restructuring. Additionally, the student may begin to recognize perfectionistic thinking, identify the discomfort it produces, and identify ways in which the perfectionistic cognitive style has been learned--and thus ways to unlearn it.

We propose that this assessment phase be limited to one or two preliminary sessions in which the primary purposes are information gathering, trust building, and an opportunity for the counselor to begin orienting the student to modification of the perfectionistic cognitive style.

Phase II: Developing Self-Awareness of Perfectionistic Thinking

The second phase of intervention is directed toward encouraging self-awareness by the student of perfectionistic thoughts through the clarification of therapeutic goals, discussion of the rationale for the intervention, and a variety of other awareness exercises.

Clarifying Expectations and Goals. Important in any short-term time-limited individual process, this stage is particularly important with the perfectionistic student in light of the tendency to approach any situation with unrealistic goals. Following the assessment session(s) and some initial clarification concerning the nature of the therapy, the student may be asked to write down what s/he hopes to achieve through the therapy experience. We sometimes use a simplified goal attainment scaling form to facilitate this task (Paritzky & Magoon 1982). We may ask the student to complete this task as a homework assignment at the close of the assessment phase previously described, allowing the therapist to observe how the student responds behaviorally to goal setting (for example, does the student procrastinate, report evaluative anxiety, become over-inclusive, and so on), and to afford the student an opportunity to think further about personal self-defeating perfectionistic tendencies between sessions. The therapist and student may then discuss the goals in light of the student's perfectionistic style. The realism of the set goals and the degree to which they are representative of perfectionistic thinking are examined.

Conveying the Rationale. We believe that students in individual therapy are likely to be more motivated and cooperative if they have a cognitive map of what is to occur in the therapy and why. The therapist should take some time during this phase to educate the student about the self-defeating nature of perfectionistic thought. Using examples from the student's own situation, the therapist may share much of the information presented in the definition section of this chapter and encourage the student to elaborate on and identify the perfectionistic elements manifested. The perfectionism scale developed by Burns (1980b) can be administered to the student, thus providing an additional stimulus for discussion and a vehicle for developing self-awareness of perfectionistic tendencies. At the close of this phase, the

student is given a copy of the Burns (1980b) article to read
for homework and is encouraged to note those portions of the
article which seem especially applicable to him/her. This
article is especially useful for acquainting the student with
the self-defeating nature of perfectionism and the cognitive
restructuring approaches which will be used in the treatment.

Encouraging Increased Self-Awareness. Discussion of the
perfectionism article often generates the opportunity for the
counselor to present a variety of other exercises that may be
helpful in encouraging awareness of the student's own perfectionistic thinking. We have generated a list of perfectionistic clichés and timely sayings, such as "If at first
you don't succeed, try, try again" and "Practice makes perfect," which most students recognize and find to be part of
the cultural ideal that may perpetuate their perfectionism.
We may ask the student to read over the list and to provide
personal real-life experience examples in which the slogan
has been self-defeating.

Ellis' A-B-C analysis of rational thought is presented
to the student and illustrated during this phase (Ellis &
Harper 1975). An example provided by the student may be used
to explain the system with an emphasis on examining the perfectionistic beliefs and resulting self-talk (point B), involved in interpreting the antecedent event (point A), and
leading to the perfectionistic reaction (point C). Cognitive
therapy techniques are introduced to help the student identify the irrational, perfectionistic beliefs and assumptions
underlying the initial self-statements (Ellis & Harper 1975);
Meichenbaum 1977). The counselor may read a list of Ellis's
unrealistic, stress-producing ideas and destructive "shoulds"
(such as "If I am not a success, I am not a worthwhile person;" "I should be on top, else I'm a flop") and ask the student to identify the ones that are operative. For homework
the student is given a "perfectionist's worksheet" on which
the A-B-Cs of situations in which perfectionistic tendencies
have been activated are recorded.

*Phase III: Retructuring Self-Defeating
Perfectionistic Thinking*

Preparation for Change. In an effort to prepare the
student for the restructuring of perfectionistic thinking, we
think it is important for the student to think about the forces that will resist change. We recognize that any long-
standing cognitive pattern is not easily dismissed, particularly when it may have been mistakenly viewed as the reason
for success. We encourage the student to discuss the benefits and costs of a perfectionistic style and to recognize
the internal and external forces resisting change, as well as

the ones promoting change. A further challenge to the overly rigid perfectionistic system is attempted by instructing the student in the "Do it Perfectly" experiment. The student is asked to identify an upcoming activity or event in which an attempt at perfect conduct will be made. This paradoxical suggestion may heighten the student's resolve to overcome the perfectionistic style. It often produces confusion that temporarily disrupts the self-defeating cognitive system. The confusion can then be overcome by introducing the student to the cognitive restructuring process.

Disputing Perfectionistic Self-Talk. It is at this point in therapy that the student is encouraged to move from the task of gaining self-awareness into a more active cognitive change strategy. We try to facilitate the student's stepping outside the cognitive set and looking analytically at the perfectionistic self-talk identified at point B in Ellis' model. Continued work with the perfectionist's worksheet allows the student to consider how self-talk encompasses the stress-producing irrational beliefs identified earlier and the cognitive errors described by Beck, Rush, Shaw, and Emery (1979). Instances of all-or-none thinking can be examined. The student may be asked to observe the environment and report on the degree to which actual "perfection" can be found. Additionally, the student may be instructed to test out a core perfectionistic assumption (Burns 1980b). For instance, s/he might test the validity of the belief "I *must* be in control at all times in order to be valued by others" by exploring this thesis with a friend.

At this point, the student can be directed to point D on the perfectionist's worksheet in which the irrational perfectionistic statements at point B must be disputed. The student is directed in developing self-statements that are more rational and that facilitate coping. These "humanizers" and "realizers" can be woven into coping self-talk that can prevent and moderate point B tendencies. Meichenbaum (1977) has outlined a number of useful approaches for effecting these kinds of cognitive changes.

A powerful technique for having students confront deeply ingrained perfectionistic mental sets is to relate these beliefs to important figures in the student's past who have influenced the perfectionistic development. The student may be instructed to write an imaginary letter to one of these individuals, refute the destructive perfectionism and enumerate the advantages of a more moderate cognitive style. The student can also be asked to engage in a dialogue with an image of this source influence through guided imagery, role play, or the "talk to the empty chair" technique.

After the student has developed some coping strategies and a more balanced perspective, carrying out an experiment

in "taking a chance" can be encouraged. An activity is
selected that was previously avoided because of the perfectionistic style and the student agrees to risk the consequences of "not being perfect." Finally, the student may be
assisted in actually deciding to do something imperfectly
in an effort to illustrate that the consequences of imperfec-
tion are not as dire as the student has supposed.

Phase IV: Termination and Continuation

The final phase important in effectively intervening with
the perfectionistic college student is directed toward gaining a sense of closure and identification of ways in which
the concepts gleaned from the treatment can continue to be
utilized. The student is reminded that the treatment was
intended to help in beginning to find ways of combatting perfectionistic thinking but this point is not likely to be the
end point of development. There is evidence that a self-
control focused treatment allows for a patient's continued
improvement after termination (Goldfried & Trier 1974). The
student may be asked to reflect on the perfectionistic clichés discussed earlier and to generate alternatives conveying
the same meaning but in a less perfectionistic manner. For
example, "a job worth doing is worth doing well" was changed
by Sara to read "a job worth doing is worth doing regardless
of how well you do."

The student can be encouraged to set up a system of self-
rewards for meeting realistic goals in order to learn to
savor successes rather than devalue them. Finally, the therapist can encourage the student to reflect on the process of
the therapy, re-take the perfectionism scale, re-examine the
goals set in the initial phase and determine the degree to
which they were met, and decide to take some concrete steps
to further control perfectionistic thinking. It may be helpful for the therapist to encourage the student to schedule a
return appointment several weeks from the final session for
a follow-up or booster session. It is also possible to initiate a support group in which students can continue to work
through their perfectionistic tendencies.

Conclusion

The university students with whom we have worked individ-
ually to restructure self-defeating perfectionistic cognitions
have uniformly responded positively to the experience. They
report that the intervention has provided them with a framework through which they can better understand themselves,
and with some useful coping strategies, overcome their
destructive perfectionistic tendencies. Most students have
specifically mentioned that they appreciate the goal-oriented

nature and structure provided in the intervention process and that they have both "learned and grown" from the experience.

We believe that the intervention ideas presented here may be useful for treating a variety of presenting problems that have previously been found difficult to treat in the college population due to the diffuse and "nondiagnosable" nature of the concern. It is our hope to stimulate further thought and ultimately empirical research in the area of intervening with the perfectionistic student. In the words used by Sara in reframing a perfectionistic cliché,

> Good, better, best
> never let it rest
> until the good is better
> and the better is *good enough.*

REFERENCES

American Psychiatric Association. *Diagnostic and Statistical Manual of Mental Disorders.* 3rd Ed. Washington, D.C.: American Psychiatric Association Publications Office, 1981.

Ansbacher, H.L. and R.R. Ansbacher. *The Individual Psychology of Alfred Adler.* New York: Harper & Row, 1956.

Barrow, J.C. and C.A. Moore. "Group Interventions with Perfectionistic Thinking." *Personnel and Guidance Journal* 61 (1983):612-615.

Beck, A.T., A.J. Rush, B.F. Shaw, and G. Emery. *Cognitive Therapy of Depression.* New York: Guilford, 1979.

Burns, D.D. *Feeling Good: The New Mood Therapy.* New York: Signet 1980a.

---. "The Perfectionist's Script for Self-Defeat." *Psychology Today* 14 (1980b):34, 37-38, 41-42, 44, 46, 50, 52.

Chickering, A.W. *Education and Identity.* San Francisco: Jossey-Bass, 1969.

Ellis, A.E. and R.A. Harper. *A New Guide to Rational Living.* North Hollywood, Calif.: Wilshire, 1975.

Friedman, M. and R. Roseman. *Type A Behavior and Your Heart.* New York: Knopf, 1974.

Goldfried, M.R. and C. Trier. "Effectiveness of Relaxation As an Active Coping Skill." *Journal of Abnormal Psychology* 83 (1974):348-355.

Hamachek, D.D. "Psychodynamics of Normal and Neurotic Perfectionism." *Psychology: A Journal of Human Behavior* 15 (1978):27-33.

Malan, D.H. *The Frontier of Brief Psychotherapy*. New York: Plenum Medical, 1976.

Mann, J. *Time-Limited Psychotherapy*. Cambridge: Harvard University Press, 1973.

Meichenbaum, D. *Cognitive Behavior Modification: An Integrative Approach*. New York: Plenum, 1977.

Paritzky, R.S. and T.M. Magoon. "Goal Attainment Scaling Models for Assessing Group Counseling." *Personnel and Guidance Journal* 60 (1982):381-384.

Rogers, C.R. *Client-Centered Therapy*. Boston: Houghton-Mifflin, 1951.

7

Issues in Psychiatric Management

W.J. Kenneth Rockwell

INTRODUCTION

When working with students some issues related to diagnosis, use of medication, and psychiatric emergencies become
highlighted. These issues will be looked at in their relationship to a basic medical model which is: Doctor evaluates
patient, makes diagnosis, and recommends intervention(s)
appropriate to the condition in question; but since the final
emphasis will be placed on practical considerations, the
model may become altered somewhat.

MAKING DIAGNOSES AND RECORDS

All of the standard psychiatric diagnoses are represented
in the student population except for moderate degrees of mental retardation, chronic organic brain syndrome with substantial impairment, and diagnoses applied only to children, but
the majority of undergraduates with a psychosocial problem
who see a professionally trained help giver do not merit a
diagnosis. These students, nevertheless, can often be helped
by techniques also used to treat illnesses. Thus they receive
treatment for nonillnesses. Two issues need to be kept in
mind here: (1) how the student perceives the implications of
being treated, that is, how that implies illness with whatever
that means for the present and the future; (2) how others
might perceive it, for example, family, friends, administrators, future employers, and what being treated implies to
them. Therefore, it behooves professionals working with students to keep in mind the implications for students of being
diagnosed and being treated. Whether or not therapists
"should" diagnose students remains a controversial issue.

This controversy will not be resolved herein but some of the issues surrounding it can be considered from two perspectives (the therapist's and the student's) and administrative ramifications.

The issues are straightforward from the therapist's point of view. In the medical model, diagnosing is most useful when it leads to specific treatment for specific diseases, such as psychoses, endogenous depressions, and recurrent anxiety states that have responded to medication, and to identification of illness states, for example, sexual disorders or personality disorders, which may best be served by continuous or intermittent treatment. The function of a therapist is to identify treatable problems and treat them, and in the exercise of this function making diagnoses is useful.

Given their general level of curiosity, the number of students who ask whether or not they have a diagnosis is astonishingly small. There are a number of possible reasons for this, all conjectural. The most likely one is that whatever students may think mental disorders consist of, and their comprehension of the concepts is naturally limited, they do not think they have one. Furthermore, if they perceive the manner of the therapist as unthreatening, they may assume that their problem is not so serious as to constitute an "illness." Conversely, if they perceive the therapist as threatening or judgmental they may not want to hear how s/he has labeled them. To students, labeling means to apply an immutable categorization, and they oppose such activity just as they oppose being told who or how or what they are by authority figures at a time in their lives when they are trying to expand their horizons and shape their own identities. Finally, one of the reasons students ask about their diagnoses relatively infrequently may be that at some level they recognize that the information would be of little use to them.

In the best of all possible worlds, records generated to help conduct treatment would never become known to exist or be used for any other purpose, and other inquiries into a person's state of mind or health would require a separate and distinct evaluation in the course of which the reasons for the evaluation and the specific questions to be addressed would be made clear to all parties in advance. Reality operates otherwise, and whereas the majority of deviations from hermetic confidentiality are facilitative of treatment, the potential for substantial harm to occur through a breach of privilege is sufficient to require constant vigilance. In any given case in which confidentiality becomes an issue there will be people who will argue that a more general welfare overrides a particular individual's need for privacy.

At the local level, privileged communications statutes may or may not apply to the discipline of a given student's therapist. University administrators are likely in general to be protective of confidentiality for the practical reason that if it becomes known (among students) that they are invading it, the source of their information, be it therapist or service, is apt to become nonfunctional. Beyond the ivied walls, seekers of information are less circumspect. All records are accessible under certain circumstances and the final arbiter of what is contained in the record is the individual therapist, students themselves being generally unaware of all the foregoing contingencies. The most conservative approach to record keeping, then, is to put into the record only nonconfidential information. At this point one reaches an impasse, since the fact of a visit, its purpose, and any intervention (and the rationale therefore) are all pieces of information that literally might not be obtainable elsewhere, and yet are essential if the record is to have any meaning. From the conservative standpoint it is possible to keep all other confidential material, that is, embarrassing content, out of a meaningful record. The extent to which a therapist will limit the record will depend on his/her perception of the extent of risk to the student. If embarrassing is defined as "what we don't want others to know about us," there is a wide range of individual variation in what is considered embarrassing. Therapists are more likely to be able to judge this with some accuracy, however, than they are able to predict who will have access to the record in the future and for what purpose, both of which are usually imponderable.

In making a record, the fact of a visit and the nature of the intervention(s) are essential pieces of information. It is in describing the purpose of the visit and the rationale for the intervention(s) that the therapist has latitude. The former can be reduced to describing affective symptomatology --basically depression, anxiety, euphoria, or apathy and/or signs of cognitive impairment and the extent of these. Finally, if a diagnosis is warranted, it is included in the rationale for intervention(s). Since all psychiatric diagnoses carry potential for harming a student from an administrative perspective, for example, with reference to future education, employment, the conservative approach to record keeping would proscribe their inclusion. However, since it has become entrenched custom to include in records a substantial amount of nonessential material, the conservative approach to record keeping is unlikely to be followed in its extreme form.

Since at any given time and place some of the foregoing conflicts in perspective may be irreconcilable, a few compromises in record keeping are offered. Record creators should keep content and their speculations and opinions to a minimum. Some therapists maintain a set of "personal notes" separate from the permanent (official) record. As to diag-

nosis, one can use extra degrees of certainty before record-
ing them. For all but the most certain of diagnoses the term
clinical impression can be used, words that are less final
and more "negotiable" if need be.

From the standpoint of what a therapist tells the students about their diagnoses, it will depend on the purpose
for which the information is imparted. When students do not
have a diagnosis it is usually reassuring to them to tell
them so, especially if they have had a number of sessions,
that is, in a sense have been "treated." When a student has
a diagnosis, it does not seem to serve much useful purpose
to tell her/him the name of the diagnostic label since it is
relatively meaningless in and of itself. A discussion of
the syndrome under consideration is more useful. This is
usually a recapitulation with some embellishments of what the
student has brought in as the presenting problem and its
presumable course in the foreseeable future. The therapist
should then attempt to shift the focus to the more important
and open-ended issues of how to manage the problem(s) in
relation to day-to-day living and/or longer-term personal
development. A student who insists on knowing what his or
her diagnosis is is seeking control either through knowledge
or through rebuttal of authority (in the latter case the
student will engage in a debate and/or demand "proof" which
cannot be given). Since at that point it is a therapeutic
issue of the student's need for control, and not one of intellectual knowledge, the information that the therapist actually gives will presumably be that which will reduce the
student's anxiety by reinforcing his or her sense of control.

MEDICATION AND THE STUDENT

Given that virtually all psychiatric diagnoses are represented in the student population, all psychoactive medications may be useful in their place in treating students.
Once this generality has been stated, two other disquieting
ones immediately come to mind which will tend to make the
physician cautious in the approach to initiating treatment
with medication and will keep the physician active in reasses-
sing the need for continuation of medication once instituted.
(1) Either by their desired effects or side effects, almost
all psychiatric medications except stimulants tend to impair
the acquisition of new cognitive material and this runs
counter to the academic enterprise. ("Recreational" drugs
in the doses used do likewise, which is a substantial reason
why they are not more popular on campuses.) (2) The known
and unknown, but possible, negative effects of long-term
medication use direct the physician to use the least medication the least often as possible in such a young population.

Student Attitudes toward Medication

Most students do not like to take psychiatric drugs. The primary issue with them is: Who or what is in control of that most highly prized organ, my brain? Since many students also read, they may be aware of the issues that concern physicians, particularly the immediate, mind-altering and obtunding effects of tranquilizers and antidepressants. Furthermore, there is the "meaning" to the student of the medication itself which often is, symbolically, "severe undifferentiated mental illness" with all the loss of control implied by that. The desire to perfect mind and body in their "natural state" (whatever that may mean to the individual) may be an additional concept running counter to use of medication. Finally, fears of becoming dependent on a substance, per se, and/or dependent on the direction of an authority figure add to the resistance to taking medications.

Practical Compromises

Given the issues outlined in the foregoing paragraphs, and these are not all-inclusive, the physician will approach with trepidation even proposing that a student take psychoactive medication. With each new prescription and every renewal the physician needs to be prepared to discuss the indications for taking it, the pros and cons of both taking or not taking it, and the implications or meaning to the student of taking medication. Nothing should be done in a routine or authoritarian manner.

First of all the physician needs to decide in his or her own mind if the anxiety engendered by the proposal of medication will more than offset any potential benefit. This is not always easy to do, given the variability in effectiveness of the medications employed. Even with a clear indication for prescription, symptoms of anxiety or depression need to be moderate to severe in order for a reduction in them through use of medication to more than offset the negative reaction to the taking of it. Specific problems arise with the use of certain medications, for example, neuroleptics and lithium. One should assume that all students read the *Physicians Desk Reference* (PDR) in which they will see the indications for these medications spelled out in such terms as "antipsychotic" and "antimanic." When prescribing one of these medications the psychiatrist can expect, sooner or later, questions or comments from the student about the diagnostic implications of being prescribed these drugs. Whether or not the psychiatrist should open up such a discussion depends on the situation, of course, but the direction of such a discussion in any event needs to be away from diagnostic labeling and toward a focus on the improvement in intellectual and social functioning that will result from the mitigation of anxiety and/or depression by use of the medication.

Proposing the use of lithium is most problematic because there is no way to hedge on the diagnostic implication and provide a face-saving alternative to the patient who needs one. "Bipolar Affective Disorder" is a label more acceptable to most people than "Manic-Depressive Disease," but the blatantly out-of-control behavior implied by the word "manic" or witnessed in relatives by potential candidates for lithium therapy is particularly unpalatable to students. Also unpalatable is the notion of indefinite or life-long maintenance on a medication. Unless the indications for embarking on lithium treatment are quite clear and s/he plans to "push" for it, the psychiatrist is better advised not to mention lithium to a student at all. In the rare event that parents or a spouse have not been involved in the proceedings by the time use of lithium is proposed, they should be brought into them at this point and their support of the treatment plan enlisted.

When prescribing neuroleptics for students with schizophrenia, the denial of the illness, resistance to taking medication, and the necessity for taking it are all issues that will need to be dealt with in detail when the diagnosis has just been made for the first time or when there has been a recurrence of the illness and medication is being reinstituted. Due to the schizophrenia-neuroleptic association, proposing the use of neuroleptics to students in whom the diagnosis is uncertain, or in conditions other than schizophrenia, may be counterproductive. The psychiatrist needs to estimate that there is a high probability of success with temporary use of these medications before even mentioning them, and then initiate a discussion in which the implications to the student are explored and the most negative connotation, that is, "permanent psychotic illness," ruled out to the extent that it can be in advance.

Taking any medication means to a student that something has happened to the mind and/or emotions over which the individual has no control and this is anathema to this population. The implication to the student of this meaning and the feelings attached thereto need to be explored when the use of medication is proposed and in this context the psychiatrist needs to educate the student about the use of the medication, its various effects, and its limitations.

The basic message to deliver when prescribing any medication is that the medication will help the student gain greater self-control over thoughts, feelings, and behavior, rather than that the medication will take control. The style used to present this message should be the one that seems most likely to make the student a collaborator in this part

of treatment. With some students the message and the collaboration can often be reinforced by inviting the student to
titrate medication levels relative to the symptom(s) the
medication is designed to counter, and this may be done by
having the student manipulate a range of doses and times.
Conversely, other students may be more comfortable with the
more traditional fixed time-dose schedule, and presumably for
them control over the taking of the medication has more significance than the perceived and fantasied actions of the medication itself.

When a student declines the use of medication or resistance is seen to mount as discussion of its use progresses,
the better part of valor is for the physician to back off and
give the student time to think about it, with or without
prescription in pocket. If symptoms have not abated in an
interval, the majority of students will return willing to try
at least a little of the drug. The implied message that the
student is coping well enough to make this decision is anxiety reducing in and of itself and it invites collaboration.
Some students who continue to decline medication may be doing
so due to the belief that only the "worst cases" need medicine, and the parallel assumption that medication is the last
resort that they would like to hold in reserve and that, if
it fails, means there is no hope of relief. It is often
worthwhile to inquire about these commonly held beliefs and
rectify them to the extent possible.

PSYCHIATRIC EMERGENCIES

Psychiatric emergencies are defined as those situations
in which a determination must be made regarding whether or
not a student is emotionally ill and is suicidal, homicidal,
or unable to care for his/her own basic needs. Even when it
is determined that none of the foregoing four conditions
prevails in an absolute sense, a student evaluated with
respect to them will often be in need of care by others. It
is precisely because of the sometime necessity of involving
others in care that it is never wise for a Service or an
individual counselor or therapist to convey the message,
publicly or privately, that all contacts with students will
be maintained absolutely confidential. That there are
exceptions to confidentiality needs to be acknowledged in
a general way, and each therapist must keep them in mind in
order to proceed quickly to involve others in a student's
care when the genuine need arises.

Management of the Student

When evaluating a student in an emergency situation the first determination a psychiatrist must make is whether or not hospitalization is mandatory. The psychiatrist must know the legal criteria for involuntary hospitalization and these vary according to jurisdiction. The need for involuntary hospitalization is a professional judgment that is made unilaterally and the determination must be made internally and unambiguously by the physician. Once hospitalization is deemed mandatory, the following steps need to be taken without the student's knowledge: (1) location of a hospital that has space immediately for a committed patient and (2) assemblage of the means for getting the student there, involuntarily if necessary.

After the above preparations have been made the psychiatrist can begin to talk with the student about the reasons why hospitalization is desirable at this time and solicit a voluntary admission. Resistance to hospitalization is the most usual immediate response, but a substantial number of students will agree after an hour or two of discussion during which time some of their initial anxiety about such a step will have abated. Among those who remain adamantly opposed, a large percentage will go voluntarily rather than be committed when those alternatives are presented. It is for the few remaining that the elaborate preliminary preparations are necessary. The guiding psychodynamic principal is that once the student has been determined to be out of control, the psychiatrist must demonstrate to the student that sufficient external controls are available to make life safe. When a clear message is given, few students are so disturbed as to be unable to receive it, and the resulting reduction in tension in the majority of them facilitates collaboration.

If the psychiatrist determines that hospitalization is not mandatory, all other management options become available and the question to be answered is: What is the least restrictive environment that will be sufficiently supportive to help diminish the symptomatology that defines the emergency? Material and psychological features of the environment are included in this assessment. The range of material options available may include residence in a hospital, infirmary, home of family of origin, with friends, or return to usual living quarters. The psychological environment is affected by changes in patterns of human contacts, patterns of activities, and the actions of medication on the internal milieu.

Psychiatrist and student may come rapidly and spontaneously to the same conclusion regarding what combination of the above factors seems appropriate to the immediate situation. More often there will be some diversity of opinion on management that will require discussion and perhaps compromise. Usually, a systematic review is necessary of all the possible combinations that might be used to help manage the situation. Such a review, conducted patiently by the psychiatrist, can serve a number of purposes. Foremost, it serves to expand the evaluation of how well the student is likely to be able to control his/her behavior and cooperate with the management plan. When the student is able to discuss options in a meaningful way, s/he is brought thereby into the decision-making process and his/her sense of control is enhanced, a factor favorable to the restoration of emotional equilibrium. Attention is directed away from causes and symptoms and toward problem solving, with the positive implication that help is forthcoming. Most students have not really reviewed within themselves all the practical alternatives and even if the visit to the psychiatrist is forced upon them, one of their hopes is that the latter will have a magical solution for the situation. They are unaware of how relatively limited and prosaic the practical options are, but when directed gently to the realities, they will often help construct, albeit reluctantly, a practical management plan. During these discussions the psychiatrist has two major sources of persuasion. S/he can compliment the student's good sense and judgment in deciding to take steps that are unpleasant but that will help resolve the situation and s/he can give repeated reassurances that the present state of affairs and the interventions needed to bring it under control are both temporary.

Criteria for voluntary hospitalization hinge on too many variables to attempt to review them fully in this chapter. When the student's degree of safety, most usually to self, is undetermined but is of serious concern to the psychiatrist and/or others, hospitalization is indicated until clarification is achieved. Potentially suicidal or otherwise acutely and severely emotionally disturbed students require the services of people professionally trained to deal with those states. Most of the resistance to the use of a psychiatric facility arises from insufficient appreciation of that fact. A few infirmaries are staffed with personnel so trained; otherwise, they are usually unavailable on a 24-hour basis outside of a hospital. When it is deemed that psychiatrically trained personnel are unnecessary, all options other than the hospital become feasible and the issue turns to what other temporary alterations need to be made in the student's living environment, daily activities, and social contacts.

Management of the Community

Management of psychiatric emergencies almost always requires the participation of people other than the service

and student. In fact, others are usually participating
before the student arrives at the service. As a consequence,
the service seeks communication about the student outside
its walls, rather than shutting communication down. When
emotional upset is great enough to require an alteration in
usual activities (that is, class or laboratory attendance) or
living place, others must be notified. The first of these
are usually parents and then administrators who must make any
necessary formal arrangements for changes in class attendance
or academic load. People who live around the student, such
as spouses, friends, residence advisors, or landpersons
usually need to be informed, even if the student's absence
is to be quite brief. Often they have been aware that something was amiss, if not actively involved in getting the
student to the service, and keeping them apprised of developments will tend to allay their anxieties and prepare them
for resumption of relations with the student.

Whether or not there is a statutory requirement, one can
say in general that technically it is best to have written
authorization from the student for all communications with
others. Practically, such a requirement is often unnecessary
and obstructive of developing appropriate communications.
Most students will give written or verbal consent within a
reasonable amount of time, and for those who do not, belabor-
ing issues of confidentiality is not an effective emergency
management tool. In short, professionals often need to proceed on their own discretion. The content of what is communicated about the student can be limited to a brief description of the symptoms, their extent, the direction of their
magnitude, if any, and the steps being taken to manage them.
Once outside communication is opened up, the service usually
receives a great deal of information useful in planning the
longer-term aspects of management, particularly information
that gives the involved therapist a perspective on the support systems available to the student.

8

Psychosomatic Illnesses

Conrad C. Fulkerson

This chapter will consider students who present to the
university mental health professional with physical or somatic
symptoms. Despite the proliferation of terms to identify
such illnesses, I retain the term *psychosomatic* since it seems
to call to mind, for most persons, the broad range of problems that I will address. Psychosomatic illnesses involve
psychological and physiological interplay to the degree that
some consideration of that interplay is necessary in formulation and treatment. These individuals seem to experience both
emotional and "body" symptoms, though the physiologic difficulty is frequently experienced to a greater degree than the
emotional discomfort. Though minimally experienced and
expressed, the emotional component is often a major element
in the overall presenting problem.

First I will address the general issue of students who
present with emotionally related physical complaints and
comment on their evaluation and treatment in the university
mental health setting. I will then consider two particular
psychosomatic illnesses, eating disorders and sleep disorders,
that occur with some regularity in university students and
about which student mental health professionals need some
particular knowledge and awareness.

THE GENERAL APPROACH TO PSYCHOSOMATIC ILLNESS

Often, the term psychosomatic illness brings to mind a
person who reports physical discomfort with a relative
absence of observable (by patient, onlooker, or physician)
evidence of any illness that could bring about the symptoms.
The concept is extraordinarily broad and could encompass anything from a tension headache, experienced by most everyone,

to possible relationships between emotions and sudden death
(Lown, DeSilva, Reich, & Murawski 1980). Closely related
concepts include the psychoanalytic idea of hysteria or conversion reaction, hypochondriasis, somatic delusions, and
the DSM III category of somatoform disorders (DSM III 1980).
While these and other terms are all slightly different, I
will, except for a brief overview of differential diagnosis,
consider them more or less together and speak primarily of
general approaches.

To bring some focus to this discussion and provide a
basis for later assessment and treatment considerations it
may be helpful to sketch three case histories that are representative of the psychosomatic problems that have presented
at Counseling and Psychological Services.

Case 1

A 23-year-old single male graduate professional school
student came to CAPS during the first two weeks of school and
reported that his personal physician had suggested that he
obtain assistance in dealing with stresses of his upcoming
academic program. The student was new to this school and had
attended college on a much smaller campus.

The student's physician had treated him for the past
three years for recurrent abdominal pain that seemed increased
at times of stress. Various tests, including x-rays, revealed
no anatomic or physiologic abnormality and the physician had
made the diagnosis of "spastic colon." A medication usually
provided relief but the student was concerned that despite
this medication the demands of the graduate program might be
too great and the pain might return and become intolerable.
After only a little further listening, the student expressed
to the therapist his concerns about performance in school
generally and his questions regarding whether he would "measure up."

Case 2

A 20-year-old woman who was in her third year of the
undergraduate nursing program came to CAPS because of anxiety
about dizziness and an obscure "heaviness" of her head. Specifically, she expressed concern that she might have a brain
tumor. She had recently seen a neurologist who advised her
that there was no detectable abnormality on examination or
tests and suggested that this might be her "nerves." The student indicated that she really did not feel any emotional
discomfort beside the concern over her symptoms and, in fact,
really did not believe that she had a brain tumor. Nevertheless, she was preoccupied with the possibility and attributed
her emotional suffering to her physical symptoms. She said
that she was not sure just what kind of doctors there were at

CAPS but that perhaps I could talk with her about her illness and make some suggestions.

Case 3

The campus student health service referred a 19-year-old single man who presented to their clinic for evaluation of a rapid, pounding heartbeat that occurred suddenly, intermittently, and without warning. At these times he felt weak and tight in his chest. The student was the youngest of several children, his father had died of heart disease when he was quite young, and the student had recently left his home locale for the first time when he stopped working and came to the university to study medical technology. This man was reluctant to come to CAPS and was puzzled that medical evaluation did not reveal some heart problem. He was equally uncertain that a psychological problem could play a role in this illness.

Each of these three students had initially sought assistance from medical physicians and out of that assessment came for psychological evaluation. Occasionally students with somatic complaints come directly for mental health services and subsequent adjunctive medical evaluation may be indicated, as I will discuss. It is important, however, to take seriously all students who present themselves even if their choice of initial professional help seems, at first, incongruous with their complaint. There is often wisdom in these choices at many levels, even unconsciously.

We have also seen a number of students coming for counseling with emotional distress stemming from specific medical illnesses. The emotional concern generated by the diagnosis of genital herpes is widely known and is an excellent example of an illness for which many sufferers have sought psychological counseling in addition to medical evaluation.

The initial evaluation of the student with psychosomatic complaints is much the same as with any student seeking brief counseling. Occasionally psychotherapists without medical training or without experience with such patients may feel intimidated or overwhelmed by the student's physical difficulties. While referral in this instance is certainly appropriate, it is possible, with some experience and collaboration with medical colleagues, for most therapists to evaluate and often to offer psychotherapy for these students. The students may focus to varying degrees on their medical ills or may, in the mental health setting, move quickly to discuss their feelings, thoughts, and worries. The basic history of medical symptoms may be obtained using the approach of Engel and Morgan (1973) which determines a symptom's bodily location, quality, degree, duration, and course since appearance, setting(s) of occurrence, aggravating and alleviating influences,

and associated manifestations. The psychologically trained
practitioner is in a particularly good position to collect
further information about the physical distress by determining the context of the symptom psychologically, interper-
sonally, and as related to psychosocial events over time.

Chronic pain syndromes have been approached with some
interesting assessment techniques (Fordyce 1976). This
approach includes learning in detail the time pattern of the
symptom, the duration, how usual activities are changed with
the symptom, and the responses that patients receive from
those around them as a consequence of the symptom. One
should include in the student's interpersonal network his
or her family since they are usually "just a phone call away."

In addition to information concerning the medical complaint, a psychiatric history is taken. The therapist
searches for connections between stresses, losses, and patterns of illness experienced by the student or family, and
the psychosomatic symptom. A careful mental status examination is important with attention to the student's mood and
evidence of the physiological or psychological indicators of
depression. All current concerns that the student expresses
are carefully explored with particular attention to concomit-
tant feelings that may be elicited by the discussion.

A brief family history is always indicated and I find
more often than not that it provides significant information.
I usually draw a simple family tree to include parents,
siblings, grandparents, or other important persons, noting
health problems, psychiatric history, and the dates of death
of any deceased persons. This is extremely useful in identifying unresolved grief, psychological identification with
family members through the symptom, a family history of
depression, and the status of relationships with important
others.

The history in psychosomatic illness is intriguing, complex, and associated with some pitfalls. The problem is,
essentially, a mystery for the sufferer, referring physician,
and student mental health therapist. Though it is presumed
by the lack of medical "findings" that there is an emotional
contribution to the symptom, and the student somewhat acknowledges this by coming for the psychological evaluation, understanding that connection and bridging that gap therapeutically
usually occurs only with considerable hard work. It is in-
cumbent upon the therapist to maintain perspective enough to
consider all data presented and, while stimulated by the
challenge that each such student presents, avoid quick determination of the "cause." It may be difficult to refrain from
voicing possibilities since most students have stumped the
physicians they have previously seen.

Any immediate impressions are working hypotheses, as in
any evaluation, and sharing such possibilities too quickly

with the student may have little beneficial effect, even if "obvious" to the therapist. The student has thus far skill-fully hidden these emotional issues from him or herself by experiencing them somatically. The resolution of psychoso-matic illnesses that prove eventually to have a conflictual or unconscious component comes only with the timely interpre-tation of that issue in the therapy process when the student is ready.

With the data gathering completed, a formulation of the problem is in order. First, one must consider the degree of physical illness vs. emotional distress that is present. Does the student seem, in fact, to have significant medical illness with marked suffering or debility? In Case 2, could we, in fact, be certain that no brain tumor was present? Even if psychological issues have been uncovered, significant remaining questions about the student's physical well-being (such as avoiding injury due to "psychosomatic fainting") should be answered by further collaboration and consultation. The therapist must be satisfied that the student is reason-ably stable and suitable for psychological treatment.

If the medical status is stable and further investiga-tions seem unwarranted at this point (and there are *always* more tests that can be done), several general diagnostic categories can be considered. The first is the classical group of psychosomatic illnesses considered by psychoanalysts to be unconscious emotional conflicts that are manifested by an abnormality in the sensory or motor nervous system. Emo-tional concerns are said to be "converted" to physical symp-toms, hence the term conversion reaction. Classical conver-sion reactions are, in fact, most often diagnosed by neurolo-gists since the physical patterns of sensory change (numbness, tingling, etc.) or motor change (weakness or paralysis) bear no resemblance to the anatomy of the nervous system. Often, however, symptoms are vague and intermittent. Cases 2 and 3 both had symptoms arising from conflicts concerning leaving home that were "converted" into physiological experiences. They might, by some, be considered conversion reactions or, by others, somatic manifestations of stress, anxiety, grief, or depression. Classical conversion reactions as described by Freud certainly occur but, in the overall context of psy-chosomatic illnesses, they are relatively rare in the "pure" form.

A second general category to consider may be grouped under symptoms resulting from stress, anxiety, and fatigue. These are myriad and their origin in stressful situations would seem self-evident. Cumulative stress, however, is de-ceptively damaging, especially in the fast-paced, competitive campus setting. Such problems have been called "psychophysio-logic" in that psychological tension is expressed physio-logically along nervous pathways to body organs and muscles.

Common manifestations are headache, neck, and back pain, and essentially everyone occasionally suffers such difficulties in one form or another.

Case 1 manifested a particularly individual reaction to stress, as noted in her presenting history, with abdominal cramping from intestinal overactivity. Other individuals with particular predispositions may have physiological reactions to stress in the forms of peptic ulcer, asthma, musculoskeletal pain, or elevated blood pressure. A particular manifestation of the stress of academic life is disordered sleep and will be considered separately. A careful evaluation of recent and current stress levels is indicated in every evaluation since both on and off campus stress is becoming recognized as a significant contributor to physical suffering.

Somatic delusions accompanying psychosis are a third category of psychosomatic illness and may move the student to seek medical help. A key characteristic of these, in addition to the probable identifiable psychosis found on the mental status examination, is their extraordinarily bizarre and frightening content. The delusional student may complain of "snakes and parasites moving through my body destroying me inside" or "fire burning in my brain." The student often reports that these seem to be actually happening rather than to be describing metaphorically a feeling or symptom. Treatment of delusions consists of treatment of the psychosis, almost always with medication, and they are mentioned here to underscore the need for recognition.

Among these general diagnostic categories none are more important than disturbed mood and the role that depression may be playing in the illness. The appreciation of childhood and adolescent depression has grown greatly in the past few years and frank depressive illness presenting as psychosomatic illness in adolescents and young adults appears to be a common occurrence (Lesse 1981). Depression is likely to occur, to some degree, in all psychosomatically ill students or may be the major factor underlying the experience of physical illness. Mood state may, in a rough analogy, be considered similar to body temperature in that it varies over time periods in a cyclic fashion, it seems to respond to both internal (thoughts or worries) and external (environmental stresses) influences, and, when abnormally depressed or elevated, mood level may interfere with functioning. The assessment of a student's spirits or feelings is as central to the psychiatric assessment as taking the temperature or pulse in the physical examination.

Case 2, described above, upon the recommendation of the referring neurologist and with the vigorous agreement of the CAPS psychiatrist, was treated with the antidepressant medication amitriptyline. With this treatment she experienced dramatic clearing of her symptoms of dizziness and "heaviness" in her head. In my experience depression plays a significant role in most psychosomatic presentations. Lesse (1981), in a report of 141 adolescents with depression presenting as psychosomatic illness, profiles the personality characteristics of these young people. They were almost uniformly considered to be "exceptional" individuals by those around them and had been excellent students. They were accomplished in leadership roles and extracurricular activities. He describes them as "meticulous, perfectionistic, overintellectualized" and remarkably sensitive to failure. Clearly, these young people were "college material." Lesse proposed a relationship between students' high expectations for achievement, the resultant stress that they placed on themselves, their depression, and their psychosomatic illness. Key in these interrelationships was their desire to retain parental respect and attention.

We have found not only depression but the adolescent issues of dependence vs. independence to be of importance in the evaluation and treatment of these young people. In hardly any other socially defined role are dependency issues so clarified as in the traditional sick role (Seigler & Osmond 1979), and at few other times of one's life are dependency issues so ambiguous as during the college years.

Intimately related to depression is a final and important consideration in this formulation, that of unresolved grief. Grief reactions are addressed in more detail in Chapter 4 of this volume. Suffice it to say that grief may be distinguished from depression by the experience of a sense of loss, while depression is characterized partly by negative thoughts about one's self that are often less prominent in grief. Occasionally grief reactions may present dramatically as psychosomatic illness when an unconscious identification with a deceased person results in symptoms or illness similar to those of the lost or deceased person. Though people experience grief from a wide variety of losses (leaving home, loss of the status experienced in secondary school, and so on), most grief associated with death may be identified through the family history, as suggested previously.

Therapists without medical training or experience may best formulate the problems of psychosomatic students by collaborating with physicians. Regrettably, not all physicians have training or interest in bridging the gap between psyche and soma and the therapist may need to do some exploration of resources to find a consultant who will collaborate beyond reporting that "all of the tests are negative." Relevant and appropriate information to obtain from a physician consulting in such cases includes the potential seriousness of the somatic complaint, specific need for periodic follow up, and some general idea regarding physiologic mechanisms that may

bring about the reported symptoms. For example, a therapist
may be better able to treat a student in psychotherapy by
understanding the mechanism by which certain symptoms are
physiological manifestations of anxiety. If possible, it is
useful for the physician to share with the therapist his/her
thinking process, in a brief step-by-step fashion, in determining that this is a psychosomatic illness.

After formulation of the basis for the complaints, treatment planning naturally follows. Whether a student with such
difficulties is a candidate for treatment in the student mental health setting is an important consideration. Agency
policy may limit sessions, appropriate consultation may not
be available as freely as desirable, or the psychological
factors operating may indicate a need for long term psychotherapy.

In addition to student and agency considerations, there
are important therapist considerations in the decision to
treat or to refer. Many therapists simply do not enjoy working with patients with medical complaints. Students with
somatic ills may attempt to place considerable responsibility
on the clinician as in the traditional sick role and medical
model. In this widely held view, it is not required that the
patient know or even seek to know what problems exist--the
"doctor" is supposed to attend to that. In psychotherapy
there is considerably more responsibility placed on the
client and if the psychosomatic student is to benefit from
counseling or therapy, some clarification and possibly some
shift in perception of just where the responsibility lies is
often necessary. These contrasting roles are well outlined
in Seigler and Osmond's *Patienthood* (1979). It is most
important that the therapist be willing to take the student's
complaints seriously and listen attentively to what may at
times seem to be an indistinguishable or confusing mix of
illness and affect (Whitaker 1981).

The importance of therapeutic relationship, central in
all psychological treatment, cannot be overestimated in
approaching psychosomatic students. Previously unsuccessful
treatment attempts may have been limited to specific techniques, whether medical (for example, medication) or psycho-
physiological (for example, biofeedback or relaxation). Valuable as these measures may be, the psychosomatic problem may
continue because it, in part, involves feelings, people, and
relationships. Effective treatment requires appropriate
human involvement by the therapist for which particular techniques cannot substitute.

The treatment of these students in the university mental
health setting is usually some form of brief psychotherapy.
Dynamic or insight-oriented psychotherapy has posed problems
both in theory and in practice when employed in psychosomatic
illness. Karasa (1979) outlines these problems well, describ-

ing both therapist and patient variables that contribute to them. One interesting (and frustrating) concept is that of alexithymia. Psychosomatic patients are seen, by some, to have marked difficulty in expressing emotions verbally (*alexithymia:* "no words for mood") and limited ability to use fantasy. Systematic research in this regard has been difficult and limited (Lesser 1981), but the concept itself offers some idea of the difficulties with this particular application of traditional dynamic therapy. Karasa underscores the importance of flexibility by the therapist and patient-therapist compatibility and relationship. He suggests initially relating to the patient as a clinician through what he terms the "health alliance," becoming thoroughly familiar with the somatic difficulties, and maintaining a close alliance with involved physicians. He then moves to develop a "life alliance" where therapist and patient deal with current areas of living besides the illness symptom. This evolution may progress to a model of treatment essentially the same as traditional psychotherapy.

I have found that the phases identified by Karasa may be traversed rather rapidly with many college students. This may be due to the brief duration of many of these illnesses, the frequent absence of an established "psychosomatic character structure" focused entirely around illness, and the basis of many of these complaints in issues of depression and dependency associated with adolescent development. Whitaker (1981) reports similar success in relatively brief psychotherapy with psychosomatic college students attained by urging them to move rather directly to deal with emotions such as anxiety or sadness. He also notes that with a good therapeutic relationship and brief therapy many presenting somatic difficulties may fade or disappear without obvious reason when the emotional issues are addressed. Proceeding rapidly to emotional issues is not contradictory to my caution about drawing connections between psychological issues and symptoms too quickly. With brief treatment, I refer to moving ahead rapidly with treatment itself, involving affective issues. The previous cautionary note was a warning against premature "intellectual" exercises that might be tempting when seeing the fascinating phenomenon of mind affecting body.

Some strategic reframing by the therapist may be helpful during early sessions. One means of doing this is to introduce the student to a "stress model" of conceptualizing their illness. Certain reference materials for assigned reading may be useful, such as *Stress, Sanity, and Survival* (Woolfolk & Richardson 1979). Also useful is the concept of the cumulative nature of stress, itemizing stresses with the student, and some general education around the relationship between stress and psychological events. Such an approach begins to build a mutually understood model for therapist and student, may help demystify the illness, and may plant the seeds of "psychological mindedness."

Once a satisfactory working relationship has been established, there are some techniques that may be adjunctively useful. Students may keep a detailed diary of their experience of the somatic difficulties. In this they record time, place, persons present, thoughts, and so on, that occur in conjunction with their symptoms (Mahoney & Arnkoff 1979). These records may be reviewed in the therapy sessions and often offer much fruitful material. A second technique is planned relaxation or meditation to lower general levels of stress and anxiety. Wolfolk and Richardson (1979) explain several methods in their useful and readable book. Both of these measures are applicable by students themselves and, along with the ongoing psychotherapy, can help give them a sense of mastery and control so important to both the psychosomatic patient and the late adolescent university student seeking a sense of self-determination.

The use of psychotropic medications may be invaluable but also may pose problems in at least two ways: First, medication is no substitute for a therapeutic relationship. We have seen students with physical complaints who have been medically evaluated and prescribed appropriate medication but who, with medication alone, have shown little improvement. It is my impression that a missing factor was the context of the therapeutic relationship. Second, some individuals with psychosomatic ills may have a propensity for medication abuse and the psychotropic medications with any abuse potential (primarily the benzodiazepines, such as diazepam) should be prescribed only with caution. Attention is similarly urged to avoid escalating to stronger and stronger pain medication in pain syndromes with a strong psychological basis.

With greater understanding of depressive disorders and their role in psychosomatic illness, it has often been found quite useful to use tricyclic antidepressant medication with these students. Not every depressed student will require or even be willing to take medication and unless the vegetative signs of depression such as weight loss and sleep disorder are prominent, these medications are not necessarily indicated early in treatment. Younger patients and out-patients may require smaller amounts of antidepressant than often recommended. I generally begin with low doses of amitriptyline or maprotiline (25 mg at bedtime) and increase the dose every three or four days to 75 mg or 100 mg at bedtime. Marked improvement in the presenting symptoms often accompanies improvement in sleep, concentration, and energy.

Two other treatment modalities are worthy of note. Group treatment of students with psychosomatic disorders may be extremely useful. Our experience with group treatment of eating disordered students (discussed in more detail below) has been rewarding. Though these groups may not provide a total treatment program, they offer a useful experience and are a unique contribution that the student mental health or counseling center may make. Second, some students with psychosomatic disorders may not be suitable for counseling center services, even on a short-term basis, and may require a traditional medical model for their treatment. For these students, knowledge of referral sources among internists or family physicians who are interested and trained to see and follow them regularly is extremely useful.

Treatment programs for psychosomatic students are characterized by nothing if not their need for careful individualization, especially when the program involves collaboration between psychotherapist and medical or psychiatric physician. Continued communication between clinicians, with the student's awareness and authorization, avoids confusion and double messages and allows a concerted and coordinated effort with frequent satisfying results.

EATING DISORDERS

A psychosomatic illness which has received much attention among university age persons and their families is the group of behavioral patterns known together as the eating disorders. This term, derived from the title of Hilde Bruch's landmark work (Bruch 1973), encompasses obesity, bulimia, and anorexia nervosa. Each of these disorders is believed to have a significant psychological basis though the manifestations are changes in body weight and/or difficulty with eating, food, and psychological body image.

Anorexia nervosa is defined as an intense fear of becoming obese, a distortion of body image (patients "feel fat" even when emaciated), weight loss of 25 percent of original body weight, and refusal to maintain body weight at or over a minimal normal weight. The sufferers are almost always female and the disorder is serious, with quoted mortality rates of from 15 to 21 percent (American Psychiatric Association 1980).

One characteristic of anorexia nervosa relevant to the university mental health professional is the denial that most anorectics express for the reality of their self-imposed starvation. Their attendance at counseling facilities is therefore relatively unlikely, even if they are urged to do so by friends, deans, family, or physicians. We find that we are as likely to see concerned roommates and friends of anorectic students as the students themselves.

The students are so reticent to present themselves that their initial evaluation must be handled with some delicacy even though the serious nature of their illness usually requires referral for long-term therapy or hospitalization. The therapist must first determine just how to establish some relationship with the student. This is something of a balancing act since these students may be as "put off" by experiencing too much caring or intimacy as by not feeling cared for enough. Whatever basis one may find for developing a relationship, such as the student's concern about studies, worries about family or others, or even how to be "better" (a central concern of anorectics), the student must be carefully cultivated to engage his/her interest and some degree of trust. In the initial evaluation, some attention (and it may have to be rather indirect due to the student's denial) should be given to the student's physiological status. The physical consequences of the anorectic emaciation represent a potential for several types of medical emergencies. An estimate of the student's weight, evidence of illness, and signs of weakness or fatigue should be made. The mental status may suggest a metabolic disorder with difficulty concentrating or remembering. Generally, however, the initial evaluation of the anorectic reveals a "peppy," attractive, energetic but remarkably thin young woman.

Referral is usually indicated, preferably to a clinician or program experienced in treatment of anorexia. In this process consultation within the counseling or student mental health center may be helpful. The treatment of anorexia is difficult enough and team approaches, even early on, may increase the likelihood of success. A staff physician, for example, can provide expertise in assessing the student's physiological status.

The second eating disorder to be briefly addressed is bulimia. This also occurs predominantly in women and is defined as recurrent eipsodes of rapidly eating large quantities of food that is often of high caloric content or is "junk food" (whatever that may mean to the student). The eating is often solitary and inconspicuous and may be followed by voluntarily induced vomiting after the binge. Weight is usually within the normal range though bulimic individuals may experience gains and losses from alternate binges and fasts. Such students are usually aware that their eating is abnormal and fear being unable to alter it. They are often depressed and are particularly self-critical following binges (American Psychiatric Association 1980).

Students with bulimia are also quite shy about reporting their problem and therapists may meet with them for several sessions or even extended periods before this problem is acknowledged. Unlike the anorectic student, however, the bulimic is acutely aware of and, in fact, often preoccupied with, her enslavement to this lifestyle.

Bulimia is probably best approached through combined behavioral and insight-oriented treatment. The former offers some self control of binging; the latter treatment requires time, patience, and training the student to think "psychologically," but this is usually well worth the effort. The issue in all of the eating disorders is not food or weight but emotions and relationships including one's relationship with one's self.

Though both behavioral and insight-oriented treatment programs may be of a long-term nature and therefore beyond the capability of the campus mental health facility, we and others have found that group approaches for students experiencing bulimic behavior can be successfully conducted on a time-limited basis within the college counseling center (Roy & Kahn 1982; Boskind-Lodahl & White 1978). Such groups provide mutual support, a setting where behavior and feelings that are perceived as painful or shameful can be acknowledged and discussed, and an opportunity to learn the basics of eating, nutrition, and weight maintenance. Beside discussion and education, some of the behavior therapy components of a multidimensional approach to bulimia may be included in these groups.

SLEEP DISORDERS

All students entering a residential college or university and participating in academic and extracurricular activities experience changes in basic living patterns including the circumstances and schedule surrounding sleep. Just as college may change eating patterns, with meals randomly occurring and often acquiring new social or psychological significance, sleep is often lost some nights for social or academic activities with attempts to make up that sleep elsewhere. The student is confronted with more opportunity and freedom than ever. Few students know, at least initially, how to set priorities or limits for themselves.

Here, as elsewhere, in the life of the developing young adult there is overlap between the stresses and changes of college life and the problems that students bring to the student mental health or counseling center. Some knowledge of sleep problems in this setting can be of great assistance to therapists.

It has been the practice in our center for several years to ask each student coming for psychosocial counseling to complete the Zung Self-Rating Anxiety and Depression Scales (Zung 1965, 1971). Both scales contain, among the 20 items on each, one item pertaining to sleep. The depression scale item is stated, "I have trouble sleeping at night" and the student is asked to indicate whether this occurs none, some, a good part, or all of the time. Similarly, on the anxiety scale the item, "I fall asleep easily and get a good night's rest," is rated on a one to four basis.

In 1982–83, 630 undergraduate, graduate, and professional school students coming to CAPS completed both sleep items on these scales. The students' ages ranged from 16 to 41 and averaged 21.4 (S.D. 3.4). Three hundred thirty-seven students (53.5 percent of the total) indicated that they experienced current sleep difficulty "a good part of the time" or "all the time" on one or both of the two items; 140 students (22.2 percent) indicated such sleep difficulty on both sleep items, and 43 students (6.8 percent) checked both items to indicate that they experienced difficulty essentially all of the time.

The sleep items on each scale correlated highly with the respective depression and anxiety scores and with most other individual items. We conclude that the majority of students who reported sleep difficulty did so in the context of anxiety, depression, or both.

In a West Coast community survey (Soldatos, Kales, & Kales 1979), 33 percent of representative householders reported current difficulty sleeping and 42 percent had either current or past complaints in this regard. The same source reported that 70 to 75 percent of psychiatric in-patient and out-patient populations have some type of sleep disturbance. Though these prevalence data and our depression and anxiety scale data use different methodology and therefore may not be exactly comparable, it is not surprising that students coming for psychosocial counseling, many of whom have transient difficulties and respond to very brief interventions, would report sleep difficulty somewhere between the general population and a more formally defined psychiatric population. The finding that over half of these students report some difficulty sleeping supports the contention that some familiarity with sleep disorders could serve the student mental health professional well.

Classifications of sleep disorders are becoming more sophisticated and an appreciation is growing for importance of the one-fifth to one-third of our lives that we spend sleeping. For purposes of evaluating sleep disorders, I will focus on some pertinent inquiries that may be made concerning sleep status and review common sleep problems with interventions that may be useful.

Though specific data are lacking, it is our impression, supported by others (Roffwarg & Altshaler 1982), that individuals experiencing sleep difficulty, especially in the setting of emotional upheaval otherwise, may be unlikely to mention sleep as a problem and this may, in part, be fostered by a lack of awareness by the examining clinicians. It is appropriate, then, in the initial interview, to at least briefly touch upon this area.

In addition to asking for the students' overall assessment of their sleep, the therapist may ask more specifically just *how* sleep is disturbed, the duration of that problem, and inquire about the sleep-wake status of the entire 24-hour period. Basically, individuals may be troubled by sleeping too little or too much. The quality of sleep may also be disturbed by awakening or other disruption, so that the sleep obtained may not, even if quantitatively "normal" for that individual, leave a rested feeling.

Hypersomnia (sleeping too much) may represent a variant of depression, though depression is usually characterized by insomnia. In particular, hypersomnia may be associated with depressed mood in adolescence. Students may also sleep more to avoid situations perceived as unpleasant, or uncomfortable thoughts or feelings. Daytime somnolence may be a presentation for otherwise unrecognized nighttime sleep difficulty. On rare occasions, episodes of rapidly and uncontrollably falling asleep during the day, sometimes associated with loss of voluntary muscle tone, may occur and suggest the specific sleep disorder, narcolepsy.

Most sleep complaints center around not enough sleep, or the insomnias. Difficulty falling asleep (initial insomnia) is most often a manifestation of stress and anxiety. Marked difficulty sleeping initially and throughout the entire night may be an early indication of psychosis. In fact, this had been a common presentation of psychosis (both affective and schizophreniform) in our center.

Difficulty remaining asleep, with or without other sleep disruption, may indicate a variety of difficulties including anxiety, depression, psychosis, or general stress or fatigue. Both initial and middle insomnia may be greatly aggravated in the college dormitory where a few students may disturb a great many others.

Drugs may adversely affect sleep and their effects are usually noted during the early and middle sleep phases. Prior use and then discontinuance of hypnotic drugs may result in "rebound" insomnia. Caffeine in beverages can easily delay sleep without the offending substance seeming implicated. Alcohol, so long used as a bedtime sedative, actually may contribute to awakening during the night as the substance is metabolized, the blood level falls, the depressant effect wanes, and a central nervous system rebound excitability results.

Awakening early in the morning, usually with a feeling of having rested poorly and/or notable dysphoria, is the classic (though not necessarily the most common) sleep disturbance of depression. This recognition, along with the extreme sleep difficulty that may herald psychosis, may provide extremely useful indicators of a student's presenting problem.

Finally, recent sleep laboratory research (Institute of Medicine 1982) has recognized some effects of "jet lag" and shift work under the category of sleep phase disorders. Suffice it to say here that any of us (not only infants) may "get our days and nights mixed up" and attempts to sleep may become out-of-phase with our internal biological rhythms that enhance falling asleep at some times and at other times make it much more difficult. The campus setting with parties, examination periods, term papers, and so on, is an environment conducive to such disturbance, that may then be perpetuated by cumulative fatigue and stress. Accompanying stimulant use to enhance performance often complicates this problem.

Several suggestions or prescriptions (behavior as well as pharmacologic) may help students with sleep disorders. Often these problems are relatively acute and situational, with a history going back only a week or ten days. The shorter the duration of the problem, the more likely that brief interventions will help. The goal in the student mental health setting is to offer suggestions about such brief disorders, identify underlying psychiatric disorders that may present with sleep difficulty, attempt to identify more serious disorders of sleep when they occur, and make appropriate referral.

Many sleep problems begin to resolve as anxiety diminishes after beginning brief psychotherapy. With brief situational disturbances, we often offer one or two nights of mild hypnotic medication such as flurazepam. This may seem at odds with much sleep literature but that literature tends to focus on more chronic varieties of insomnia. Since students may benefit from "resetting" their sleep cycle in this way, it seems appropriate to maintain a supply of such a medication at the center in order to dispense small amounts when indicated. This is greatly appreciated by students and avoids their having to fill a prescription for one or two tablets. Adequate precautions and record keeping must, of course, be maintained.

Though insomniacs may attribute their sleep difficulty to the environment more than is warranted (by contrast, others in the same environment seem to sleep well), the campus living environment is often not conducive to regular sleep despite the best efforts of the institution. Information should be obtained in the history about living conditions, such as number of roommates, dorm character and location, and so on. We have effectively addressed problems of this type by advising students about assertion and negotiation with those around them to bring their living circumstances more into line with their psychological, social, and physical needs.

Though sleep disorders may improve quickly with brief counseling and coordinating schedules or establishing quiet times, many students benefit from further advice. Principles of "sleep hygiene" include: regular retiring and awakening, avoiding caffeine and alcohol (especially late in the day), moderating exercise and exercising early in the day, having

a quiet, relaxing "wind down" time, not staying in bed when
sleep is difficult but going elsewhere and quietly reading
something enjoyable until sleepy, and moderating eating before
retiring (Roffwarg & Altshaler 1982). Even though these may
sound like tips from a junior high health class and perhaps
not appeal to "independent" undergraduates with their emerging
sophistication, they all have definite and, in fact, rather
complex physiologic bases. Students may find some of these
ideas more acceptable when framed as findings of research,
and implications of some of the mechanisms are explained such
as the effects of alcohol on sleep and the need to coordinate
sleep time with natural, internal rhythms.

Besides the indications for the brief use of benzodiazepine hypnotics, significant depression with many physical
features and, certainly, psychosis are indications for pharmacologic intervention. Many centers will want either to
hospitalize or refer psychotic students, though this is not
always necessary. In any event, medication for psychosis is
essentially always indicated.

Drug treatment of depression is somewhat less clear-cut
and varies with individual students, the therapist's orientation and training, and the availability of psychiatric con-
sultants. When antidepressant medication is used for depression with associated insomnia, the more sedative drugs of
this group such as amitriptyline or maprotiline are most useful. The sleep disorder and anxiety component of depression
may be so severe initially that additional small amounts of
benzodiazepine may be useful for a few days to two weeks.

Profound fatigue and/or sleep phase disorders can debili-
tate students. Brief admission to the campus infirmary for
one to three days can be extraordinarily useful to allow them
to readjust their sleep-wake cycle, generally rest, and re-
cover in a quiet environment. When this is coordinated with
the infirmary staff and all involved understand the simple
goals of the stay, the restoration possible is often dramatic.

Two particular sleep disorders, formerly thought to be
exotic and unusual but which are being recognized more often,
are narcolepsy and sleep apnea. They are noted here for com-
pleteness and to increase awareness of such problems occurring in university students. Referral is usually indicated.
Narcolepsy, as already noted, is a disorder in which sudden-
onset sleep occurs in the daytime during inactive periods or
the sleep is triggered by laughing or emotion. The episodes
last a few seconds to several minutes and usually leave the
individual feeling refreshed with no memory of the incident.
They may be accompanied by loss of muscle tone or falling.
Since narcolepsy usually begins in the late teens or early
twenties, students with the disorder may certainly present to
college mental health centers. Sleep apnea is a syndrome of
cessation of breathing during sleep that may cause awakening

and therefore present as insomnia. The episode is often unrecognized by the individual, who is usually a snorer. Occasionally, daytime sleepiness is a complaint. The diagnosis by history is more difficult than with narcolepsy and may require data from a roommate or bed partner or sleep laboratory observation.

In summary, inquiry into sleep status can be of benefit to students coming to the university mental health professional. Greater understanding of the student's overall functional level, assistance in dealing with acute stress and fatigue syndromes, and clues to some serious psychiatric disturbances can be gained. With restoration of sleep patterns through general reduction of anxiety, using brief psychotherapy, brief administration of hypnotic medication, specific treatment of psychiatric disorders, or recovery from fatigue induced by a disordered sleep-wake cycle, students can better cope with the demands of campus life and move onward in their academic pursuits.

REFERENCES

American Psychiatric Association. *Diagnostic and Statistical Manual of Mental Disorders*. Washington, D.C.: American Psychiatric Association, 1980.

Boskind-Lodahl, M. and W.C. White, Jr. "The Definition and Treatment of Bulimarexia in College Women--A Pilot Study." *Journal of the American College Health Association* 27 (1978):84-87.

Bruch, H. *Eating Disorders*. New York: Basic Books, 1973.

---. *The Golden Cage*. New York: Vintage Books, 1979.

Engel, G.L. and W.L. Morgan. *Interviewing the Patient*. London: W. B. Saunders, 1973.

Fordyce, W.E. *Behavioral Methods for Chronic Pain and Illness*. St. Louis: C. V. Mosby, 1976.

Institute of Medicine. "Sleep, Biological Clocks, and Health." In *Health and Behavior*, edited by D.A. Hamburg, G.R. Elliott, and D.L. Parron. Washington, D.C.: National Academy Press, 1982.

Karasa, T.B. "Psychotherapy of the Psychosomatic Patient." *American Journal of Psychotherapy* 33 (1979):354-364.

Lesse, S. "Hypochondriacal and Psychosomatic Disorders Masking Depression in Adolescents." *American Journal of Psychotherapy* 35 (1981):356-367.

Lesser, I.M. "A Review of the Alexithymia Concept." *Psychosomatic Medicine* 43 (1981):531-543.

Lown, B., R.A. DeSilva, P. Reich, and B.J. Murawski. "Psychophysiologic Factors in Sudden Cardiac Death." *American Journal of Psychiatry* 137 (1980):1325-1335.

Mahoney, M.J. and D.B. Arnkoff. "Self Management." In *Behavioral Medicine: Theory and Practice*, edited by O.F. Pomerleau and J.P. Brady. Baltimore: Williams and Wilkins, 1979.

Roffwarg, H.P. and K.Z. Altshaler. "The Diagnosis of Sleep Disorders." In *Eating, Sleeping, and Sexuality*, edited by M.R. Zales. New York: Brunner Mazel, 1982.

Roy, E. and E. Kahn. Personal communication, 1982.

Seigler, M. and H. Osmond. *Patienthood*. New York: Macmillan, 1979.

Soldatos, C.R., A. Kales, and J.D. Kales. "Management of Insomnia." *Annual Review of Medicine* 30 (1979):301-312.

Whitaker, L. "Interdisciplinary Considerations in the Psychotherapy of Psychosomatic Patients." *Journal of the American College Health Association* 29 (1981):236-240.

Woolfolk, R.L. and F.C. Richardson. *Stress, Sanity, and Survival*. New York: Signet, 1979.

Zung, W.W.K. "A Self-Rating Depression Scale." *Archives of General Psychiatry* 12 (1965):63-70.

---. "A Rating Instrument for Anxiety Disorders." *Psychosomatics* 12 (1971):371-379.

9

What Components of Counseling Work Best with Whom and When: A Study

Joseph E. Talley, Elinor T. Roy, and Jane Clark Moorman

How to best tailor the psychotherapeutic approach to a specific individual appears to be the primary dilemma currently facing psychotherapists in light of Bergin and Garfield's (1978) analysis of the literature. Obviously some criterion of "success" with regard to the outcome of psychotherapy must be adopted in order to investigate which components of psychotherapy are most beneficial with a specific population. However, the question regarding the components of "successful" treatment is usually raised in a manner implying that certain elements or components of therapy are efficacious with all people in all situations.

In this chapter we examine some of the commonly employed components of counseling (brief psychotherapy) in order to ascertain whether different groups of students respond to these components in different ways. In short, "What works best with whom and when?" Although this question, discussed quite thoroughly by Bergin and Garfield (1978), is not new, the conclusions of our study do offer empirically validated guidelines concerning the use of specific components for successful treatment with certain groups of students.

Given the options available as criteria for successful outcome (psychometric measurement, therapist evaluation, patient evaluation, third party observation, and so on), and the limitations of each, we adopted student satisfaction as our primary criterion. Nevertheless, we also collected self evaluations, both pretreatment and posttreatment, utilizing the Zung Self-Rating Depression Scale and the Zung Self-Rating Anxiety Scale for comparison with student ratings of satisfaction and various components of counseling.

The selection of student satisfaction as a criterion is supported by the work of Hans Strupp (1973), who utilizes patient evaluation extensively, and Horenstein, Houston, and

Holmes (1973), who found that patient evaluations of therapy were highly related to the evaluations made by independent judges, whereas therapist evaluations were not. Finally, Bergin and Garfield (1978) conclude that this criterion is as valid as any for measuring outcome.

RELEVANT LITERATURE

The early attention to client satisfaction and the client's perception of the counselor grew out of Carl Rogers' (1951) model of Client Centered Therapy. Rogers clearly emphasized that treatment would be effective if the client felt the therapist was genuine and created an environment of warmth, empathy, and "unconditional positive regard." Consequently, the Rogerian School, particularly Carkhuff, Truax, and Wargo, conducted many studies attempting to confirm the necessity, if not the sufficiency, of these ingredients as perceived by the client. Although many instruments have been developed over the years to measure client satisfaction, few have been published. One of the more utilized of these inventories is the *Counseling Evaluation Inventory* (CEI) by Linden, Stone, and Shertzer (1965). The CEI was well developed and tested regarding validity and reliability, however, such instruments become quickly dated for use as research tools since new hypotheses must be generated and tested continually. Bergin and Garfield (1978) find that no one instrument appears superior since there are a number of opinions regarding what the criteria of client satisfaction should be (for example, feeling accepted by the counselor, symptom removal, or increased insight).

Another well developed instrument is the *Psychotherapy Questionnaire, Patient Form* (PQP), utilized by Hans Strupp (1969). It has been suggested by Kline, Adrian, and Spevak (1974) that the main variable influencing client satisfaction is the degree to which the therapist is perceived as being interested in the client. It has been found that patients who were "very satisfied" with therapy described their therapists as warmer and more active than did patients who were "not very satisfied" (Bent, Putnam, Kiesler, & Nowicki 1976).

Considering client satisfaction in the university population, there are some established points worth remembering. Jansen and Aldrich (1973) found that patients under 30 gave significantly more negative evaluations of treatment than patients over 30 did, and Newton and Caple (1974) concluded that students seeking vocational or educational counseling were more likely to be less satisfied with services than those presenting with other concerns. Obviously, these findings are important regarding the results of client satisfaction studies conducted with students. Some studies of student satisfaction have been done to evaluate the efficacy of brief psychotherapy in the campus environment. Weber and Tilley (1981) concluded that approximately 80 percent of presenting students could benefit from a brief therapy format. Resnick (1978) has addressed the need to know what subpopulations of students are most satisfied.

In 1968 Stanley Strong conceptualized counseling as an interpersonal influence process, and thus counselor variables related to the ability to influence became a focus for many subsequent studies. In keeping with the interpersonal influence model, Heppner and Heesacker (1983) examined, among other things, the relationship between client satisfaction and the client's perception of the counselor's attractiveness, trustworthiness, and expertise. Although a positive relationship was found, these three variables accounted for less than half of the variance on client satisfaction ratings. (Additional literature on client satisfaction is reviewed in Chapters 1 and 3).

Considering this literature, it appeared that a client satisfaction study comparing subgroups of students (especially by sex and age) and also examining certain possible correlates of satisfaction, needed to be done. We were interested in how the interpersonal influence variable of perceived counselor expertise, some of the Rogerian relationship factors, and other technique-related variables might correlate with satisfaction.

The Zung Self-Rating Depression Scale (Appendix A, items 1-20) and the Zung Self-Rating Anxiety Scale (Appendix A, items 21-40) were selected for utilization to give additional pre- and post-treatment data. These scales have been well researched (Zung 1965; Zung, Richards, & Short 1965; and Zung 1971), are easily scored, and normative data exist for several levels of clinical severity.

PROCEDURE

The name of every other student in our card file who had come to the service for psychosocial counseling or psychotherapy during the preceding semester and was no longer receiving treatment was selected as the sample (N = 150). Of this group, those students who began treatment after the first of July (N = 49) had taken the Zung Self-Rating Scales on intake, as did all students who presented after that date with psychosocial concerns. The students in the selected group (N = 150) were sent a Client Satisfaction (evaluation-of-services) Questionnaire (Appendix B), a set of Zung Scales for a current self-evaluation and a cover letter explaining the project as necessary for the agency to evaluate its services. The students were told that the information would be kept confidential but that the responses were not anonymous since materials were numbered in order to match them with the intake data. This allowed group comparisons on the basis of sex, age, and number of sessions attended to be made.

A follow-up letter was sent to all students who did not respond encouraging them to return the forms. Those who still did not return the questionnaires after the follow-up letter were telephoned and offered new copies of the materials.

A return rate of 67 percent was achieved (N = 89), excluding letters returned undelivered and forms that were unscoreable although returned. Eight subjects were dropped from the analysis because they came for consultation about a friend or to acquire a letter to their insurance company recommending intensive psychotherapy. The remaining group (N = 81) was comprised of 53 women and 28 men. Of these students, 41 attended between one and three counseling sessions, 16 attended between four and six sessions, 10 attended seven to nine sessions, four attended 10 to 12 sessions and 10 students attended between 13 and 78 sessions. The mean age of the women was 20.78 years and of the men 23.51 years. The mean number of sessions attended by women was 8.54, while men attended a mean of 5.46 sessions.

The distribution of the sample described here is comparable in age, sex, and number of sessions attended to our total presenting population. The results of this investigation are informative in addressing three different areas. The first area of examination includes the relationship of various components of counseling and perceptions about outcome to satisfaction with services received. The second area of study is the relationship of satisfaction with services and other variables on the satisfaction questionnaire to change in anxiety and depression as measured by the Zung Scales. Finally, the data related to satisfaction and its correlates will be presented by categories of the variables of age, sex, and number of sessions attended.

RESULTS AND DISCUSSION FOR
ALL STUDENTS COMBINED

The mean ratings and standard deviations for each item of the CAPS Client Satisfaction Questionnaire, the Spearman correlation coefficients of each item with satisfaction (item 16), and the associated probability of the occurrence of each correlation under the null hypothesis are presented in Table 9.1. The variable "SATIS," the last item in the column of mean ratings, indicates the percentage of subjects who found it at least "quite true" (a rating of seven or higher) that they were satisfied with the services received (in this case

Table 9.1 Mean Ratings and Standard Deviations on CAPS Client Satisfaction Questionnaire Items for All Students Combined (N = 81) and Spearman Correlation Coefficients of All Items with Satisfaction and Associated Probability Values

Item/ Question	Mean Rating	Standard Deviation	Correlation Coefficient / Probability	
QUEST16	7.58024691	2.20150061		
QUEST1	5.90123457	2.46274714	0.62628	0.0001
QUEST2	6.19753086	2.20465277	0.73584	0.0001
QUEST3	6.70370370	2.28278582	0.74351	0.0001
QUEST4	7.09876543	2.35374668	0.68596	0.0001
QUEST5	8.07407407	1.97975868	0.68981	0.0001
QUEST6	5.82716049	2.83191686	0.50149	0.0001
QUEST7	6.33333333	2.63628527	0.75884	0.0001
QUEST8	6.22222222	2.36643191	0.54839	0.0001
QUEST9	7.79012346	2.40684466	0.66258	0.0001
QUEST10	7.70370370	1.97132217	0.70833	0.0001
QUEST11	5.92592593	2.89155057	0.47355	0.0001
QUEST12	5.27160494	2.65524173	0.51372	0.0001
QUEST13	5.12345679	3.22638620	0.18865	0.0917
QUEST14	6.43209877	2.92377441	0.01494	0.8947
QUEST15	7.72839506	1.99381760	0.74830	0.0001
SATIS	0.72839506	0.44755853	0.82165	0.0001

73 percent of all subjects). The variable "SATIS" at the bottom of the column of correlation coefficients indicates the correlation between all satisfaction ratings and those ratings that were seven or higher.

The results from questions 17, 18, and 19 on the Satisfaction Questionnaire indicated that of the total sample, 18 percent sought additional service elsewhere later, 56 percent reported that their academic performance was the same after counseling as before, 32 percent said it was better, and 11 percent worse. Forty-four percent of these studetns said the quality of their relationships with others was the same after counseling, 52 percent reported the quality to be better, and 4 percent worse. Our investigation shows that some persons do report a "deterioration effect" from psychotherapy as do most studies that inquire about it (Bergin & Garfield 1978). Obviously, deterioration is not necessarily related to counseling alone and may be influenced by many environmental and endogenous factors.

In looking at the Client Satisfaction Questionnaire, three categories relating to treatment issues are apparent, specifically, counselor-related components, process or technique-related components, and components related to outcome perception. It is evident from the correlations and probability values that all variables except feeling "uncomfortable" at times (item 14) and relating "current concerns to past family experiences" (item 13) were found to have a highly significant positive correlation with satisfaction. Nevertheless relating familial experiences to present concerns did have a modest but positive correlation with satisfaction.

The counselor and technique components most related to satisfaction were the client's feeling that the counselor was skilled, understanding, helped in clarifying what was wanted from counseling, and was encouraging. The student's feeling that "I accomplished what I had hoped to by coming to CAPS" was the item most highly correlated with satisfaction. This item, emphasizing what the student wanted, may also emphasize the role the student feels s/he played in the counseling process, as contrasted to item 15 emphasizing the counselor's expertise. Thus, despite the fact that counselor skill had a higher mean rating than did "accomplishing what I had hoped for," the latter was more positively correlated with satisfaction. This being the case, students seeing themselves as having accomplished what they themselves had hoped to appears to be a more significant correlate of satisfaction than does seeing the counselor as skilled. Further, "accomplishing what I had hope to" focuses on the total finished product rather than just counselor skill or services received. One interpretation of this finding is that more effective treatment might leave the student feeling slightly more responsible for the results of treatment than the service provider. Of course, this may be just a case of correlating two items that ask essentially the same thing.

The counselor-related correlations suggest that counselors should appear understanding, authentic, and warm (in keeping with Rogerian Theory). Yet, in agreement with the interpersonal influence model, it also appears that the counselor should be perceived as skilled and able to allow the student to feel comfortable.

Considering process or technique-related components, the data suggest that assisting the student in the clarification of what is wanted from counseling is most highly associated with positive outcome as measured by satisfaction. Encour-

aging the student to believe that the situation can improve
is another of the factors most related to satisfaction.
Assisting in the clarification of how the student has been
dealing with frustration and helping to break the problem
down into smaller parts are likewise highly related to feeling satisfied. When viewing the results of all students
together, encouraging the student to relate present concerns
to past family experiences appears to have a very modest
positive correlation with satisfaction, and having the student feel uncomfortable at times appears unlikely to enhance
satisfaction.

Thus, in going beyond client-centered relationship variables, interventions that have the greatest correlation with
satisfaction for the group as a whole are of a cognitive
nature (that is, clarification and encouragement). Psychodynamic interventions, such as relating current events to
historical family material or allowing discomfort to occur
(perhaps due to discussing problematic family material,
exploring unacceptable sexual or aggressive feelings, or
protracted silences) appear less likely to be associated with
satisfaction. Of course, this takes into account only two
psychodynamically related items and viewing the data as a
whole does not allow for individual or even group differences.
Therefore, breaking the data down for group comparisons
should make the results more meaningful.

PRE- AND POST-TREATMENT ANXIETY
AND DEPRESSION SCORES

Of the 81 students whose responses were studied, 49 began
counseling after the Zung measures were instituted as a part
of the intake procedure and thus they completed the Zung
Anxiety and Depression Self-Rating Scales both pre- and post-
treatment. The post-test raw score was subtracted from the
pre-test raw score for depression and for anxiety for each
student resulting in difference scores for both variables.
The students' depression and anxiety difference scores were
then correlated with the ratings of the items on the Client
Satisfaction Questionnaire.

Raw scores on the Zung measures may range from 20 to 80.
The mean raw score for depression on intake was 39.49, the
mean post-treatment raw score was 33.96. Although this
represents an improvement of 5.53 ($t = 4.14$, p. < .0001), mean
intake and post-treatment scores are both in the range typical of persons with Transient Situational Adjustment Reactions, Personality Disorders, or Anxiety Reactions. Regarding
the anxiety measures, the mean intake raw score was 38.39, a
score indicative of the presence of minimal to moderate anxiety. The mean post-treatment anxiety score was 31.71, indi-

cating that a difference score of 6.68 ($t = 6.02$, p. < .0001) was achieved, and the post-treatment mean anxiety score was within the normal range.

Satisfaction with services received was slightly but not significantly (p. > .05) correlated with change as measured by the Zung Scales (rho = .16850, p = .2471 for depression and rho = .13437, p = .3573 for anxiety). However, increased self understanding as rated by students was significantly related to change on both the depression and anxiety measures (rho = .37722, p = .0075 for depression and rho = .36859, p = .0092 for anxiety), as was "accomplishing what I had hoped to" (rho = .32995, p = .0206 for depression and rho = .34416, p = .0155 for anxiety). Reported change in methods of dealing with problems was quite significantly related to improvement on the depression measure (rho = .30450, p = .0334), but less so on the anxiety measure (rho = .24318, p = .0922). No other items on the Client Satisfaction Questionnaire were significantly (p. < .05) related to difference scores using the Zung Scales. Nevertheless, increased confidence in decision-making ability was highly correlated in the positive direction with change as measured by the difference scores for depressed students (rho = .27187, p = .0588).

One interpretation of the modest agreement between the Zung measures and the Client Satisfaction Questionnaire might be that as outcome measures, one of the two must be of limited validity. Although this may be the case, Bergin and Garfield (1978) have noted that different outcome measures need not always agree as they may be measuring different aspects of a multifaceted process. According to this data, depression did not show quite as much improvement as did anxiety in response to brief treatment, although the changes for both were highly significant. Nevertheless, reported decreases in depression were more associated with higher ratings on satisfaction, increased confidence in decision-making ability, increased self-awareness, and changes in methods of dealing with problems than were reported decreases in anxiety.

COMPARISONS OF THE COMPONENTS OF COUNSELING BY SEX

The responses to questions 17, 18, and 19 indicated that 21 percent of the males receiving services sought subsequent treatment elsewhere, whereas only 17 percent of the females went for additional treatment. Forty-three percent of all men reported that their academic performance was better after coming for treatment, 7 percent reported performing worse, and 50 percent of the men indicated that their performance was the same. In contrast, 26 percent of the women felt their academic performance was better, 13 percent worse, and 58 percent the same. (Approximately 3 percent of the women did not respond to this item.) Thus, men were much more likely than women to report improved academic performance after counseling.

With regard to the quality of relationships with others, 54 percent of all men found the quality to be better after treatment, 7 percent reported the quality as worse, and 39 percent indicated that the quality was the same. Fifty-one percent of all women felt the quality of their relationships with others was better after coming for counseling, 2 percent found the quality of their relationships to be worse, and 47 percent reported the quality of their relationships with others to be the same. The difference between the percentage of men and women reporting "worse" relationships is noteworthy but the most notable difference is that considerably more men reported that their academic performance was better after counseling. The mean ratings and standard deviations for items 1 through 16 on the Client Satisfaction Questionnaire by men and by women are presented in Table 9.2. The correlation coefficients of all items with satisfaction and the associated probability values are presented in Table 9.3.

Table 9.2 Mean Ratings and Standard Deviations on CAPS Client Satisfaction Questionnaire by Sex

Item	Females (N = 53)		Males (N = 28)	
	Mean Rating	Standard Deviation	Mean Rating	Standard Deviation
QUEST16	7.45283019	2.29184302	7.82142857	2.03767426
QUEST1	5.83018868	2.48639258	6.03571429	2.45676907
QUEST2	6.18867925	2.15778201	6.21428571	2.33106466
QUEST3	6.54716981	2.44608036	7.00000000	1.94365063
QUEST4	6.98113208	2.55320738	7.32142857	1.94467119
QUEST5	8.00000000	2.22745111	8.21428571	1.42353610
QUEST6	6.07547170	2.87461741	5.35714286	2.73812974
QUEST7	6.13207547	2.65328342	6.71428571	2.60849244
QUEST8	6.33962264	2.41743186	6.00000000	2.29330749
QUEST9	7.67924528	2.76498425	8.00000000	1.53960072
QUEST10	7.79245283	2.14259450	7.53571429	1.62120538
QUEST11	6.00000000	2.66024869	5.78571429	2.79360570
QUEST12	5.45283019	2.63530788	4.92857143	2.70703571
QUEST13	5.22641509	3.26191019	4.92857143	3.20795968
QUEST14	6.83018868	2.96606349	5.67857143	2.73585500
QUEST15	7.83018868	2.00706300	7.53571429	1.99038695
SATIS	0.71698113	0.45477630	0.75000000	0.44095855

Table 9.3 Spearman Correlation Coefficients of CAPS Client
Satisfaction Questionnaire Items with Satisfaction and
Associated Probability Values by Sex

Item	Females (N = 53)		Males (N = 28)	
QUEST1	0.58409	0.0001	0.71896	0.0001
QUEST2	0.73680	0.0001	0.74910	0.0001
QUEST3	0.74737	0.0001	0.72942	0.0001
QUEST4	0.72122	0.0001	0.58517	0.0011
QUEST5	0.70821	0.0001	0.65210	0.0002
QUEST6	0.57851	0.0001	0.37695	0.0480
QUEST7	0.73632	0.0001	0.80531	0.0001
QUEST8	0.53401	0.0001	0.61028	0.0006
QUEST9	0.64245	0.0001	0.79098	0.0001
QUEST10	0.76360	0.0001	0.59061	0.0009
QUEST11	0.42897	0.0014	0.58511	0.0011
QUEST12	0.50350	0.0001	0.57504	0.0014
QUEST13	0.06062	0.6663	0.48525	0.0089
QUEST14	−0.07334	0.6017	0.27499	0.1567
QUEST15	0.75284	0.0001	0.77328	0.0001
SATIS	0.80800	0.0001	0.85531	0.0001

Mean ratings indicate a slightly higher satisfaction rating
by men than women, and 75 percent of all men rated the satisfaction item as at least "quite true" while 71 percent of
women did so; however, the mean satisfaction ratings are not
appreciably different.

Looking at the correlation of satisfaction with various
components of psychotherapy grouped by sex, some differences
are evident. For males, all components of counseling represented by items 1 through 15, with the exception of feeling
uncomfortable at times (item 14), were significantly ($p = <$
.05) correlated with satisfaction, including the exploration
of current events as related to past familial experiences
(item 13). Although feeling uncomfortable at times was not
significantly correlated with satisfaction, the relationship
between the two items was positive. The most important (as
evidenced by the correlation with satisfaction) counselor
components for males were perceived counselor warmth and

skill (items 9 and 15). The outcome variable, "I accomplished what I had hoped to by coming to CAPS," was extremely high in its association with satisfaction for men and the most important technique-related component was clarifying what was wanted from counseling (item 2).

The females differed from the males in that feeling uncomfortable at times was negatively correlated with satisfaction, and relating current situations to past family experiences showed almost no relationship to satisfaction. Perceived counselor skill was a little less important (less related to satisfaction) for women than men and counselor warmth was quite a bit less important for women than for men, whereas encouragement by the counselor (item 10) was considerably more related to satisfaction for women than men. Correspondingly, feeling comfortable with the counselor (item 4) was notably more associated with satisfaction for women than men, and counselor authenticity (item 5) was somewhat more important for women than men but it was highly correlated with satisfaction for both sexes. Counselor-assisted clarification of how the student had been dealing with frustration (item 6) was found to be considerably more associated with satisfaction for women than men, and having the counselor assist in breaking the problem down into smaller parts (item 8) was less associated with satisfaction for women than it was for men.

In terms of outcome-related components, for women satisfaction was less related to perceiving that their methods of dealing with problems had changed (item 11) than it was for men, and having increased confidence in decision-making ability (item 12) was slightly less related to satisfaction for women than for men. This was also the case for increased self-understanding (item 1) though this difference was greater. Men reported (mean rating) feeling more understood by the counselor (item 3) than women, but the correlations with satisfaction were not remarkably different.

Initially it is tempting to work out explanations of the data based on the idea that students respond within the bounds of what seems to be acceptable sex-typed behavior, noting that perhaps women are more able than men to accept encouragement (item 10) and acknowledge frustration (item 6). However, this proves to be a specious explanation whenever the mean rating by one sex is higher than that of the other, but the correlation with satisfaction is nevertheless greater for the sex with the lower mean rating. Then the conclusion must be that the particular item is more valued (as evidenced by the correlation with satisfaction) by the sex with the higher correlation. For example, men reported feeling more comfortable with the counselor (item 4), but the correlation between comfort and satisfaction was greater for women. Thus, although men perceived more comfort, it appears to be more

valued by women. Hence, ratings congruent with self-image
cannot account for all differences. It appears that, just as
men and women report conditions after counseling regarding
academic work and relationships with others somewhat differently, so too, each sex to some extent may find different
elements of counseling most helpful.

Thus, from our data it would appear that in working with
male students it is most important for the counselor to be
seen as warm and skilled and assist in goal clarification.
When working with female students the data indicate that it
is most important to be encouraging, to appear skilled and
understanding, while maintaining comfort. The most important
differences concern the negative correlation between discomfort and satisfaction for women and the greater association
between relating current concerns to past family experience
and satisfaction for men. Beside these differences, all components were highly correlated with satisfaction for both
sexes.

COMPARISONS OF THE COMPONENTS
OF COUNSELING BY AGE

Mean ratings and standard deviations of three age groups
are presented in Table 9.4. (Two subjects did not indicate
an age, hence the total is less than 81.) The progressive
increase in satisfaction as age increases is consistent with
other findings noted in the literature. A gradient of the
same type (an increased rating with increased age) exists
with regard to feeling comfortable with the counselor (item
4) as well as with perceived counselor warmth (item 9). Perceived counselor authenticity (item 5) increased markedly in
the last category; however, the relationship between age and
the ratings on other items does not appear to be linear.
Sixty-eight percent of students 19 and younger found themselves to be at least "quite" satisfied with the services
received while 72 percent of the students between 20 and 22
years old reported likewise and 84 percent of those 23 years
of age or older were at least "quite" satisfied. This underscores that satisfaction is definitely related to age and
that younger students are less likely to be satisfied with
services received than older students.

Further, the responses to question 17 indicated that 20
percent of those students 23 and older sought subsequent
treatment elsewhere while 18 percent of those between 20 and
22 did so and 15.5 percent of students 19 and younger sought
subsequent treatment. Thus, it appears that older students
are more likely to seek further treatment than younger students. There were no remarkable differences by age alone for
the reported improvement of academic performance or social

Table 9.4 Mean Ratings and Standard Deviations on CAPS Client Satisfaction Questionnaire Items by Age

Item	19 and Younger (N = 32)		20-22 Years Old (N = 22)		23 and Older (N = 25)	
	Mean Rating	Standard Deviation	Mean Rating	Standard Deviation	Mean Rating	Standard Deviation
QUEST16	7.43750000	2.19878999	7.81818182	2.32248561	7.92000000	1.77763888
QUEST1	5.68750000	2.70528157	6.18181818	2.42283509	6.16000000	2.09523268
QUEST2	6.34375000	1.97744336	6.00000000	2.26778684	6.48000000	2.31156513
QUEST3	6.71875000	2.17366014	6.50000000	2.34520788	7.20000000	2.16024690
QUEST4	6.71875000	2.30335485	7.09090909	2.75869346	7.76000000	1.98494332
QUEST5	7.90625000	2.20497056	7.90909091	2.34843597	8.60000000	1.08012345
QUEST6	5.68750000	3.11538844	5.59090909	3.09622029	6.48000000	2.08406654
QUEST7	6.25000000	2.92927383	6.81818182	2.38320240	6.20000000	2.46644143
QUEST8	6.46875000	2.62720721	6.04545455	2.14869335	6.36000000	2.09920620
QUEST9	7.40625000	2.46078109	8.13636364	2.98081891	8.16000000	1.67531092
QUEST10	7.53125000	2.06326354	8.13636364	2.07698166	7.72000000	1.69607390
QUEST11	6.43750000	2.47487373	5.40909091	3.24637660	5.92000000	2.32594067
QUEST12	5.37500000	2.69707129	5.40909091	2.68433003	5.16000000	2.64070698
QUEST13	4.81250000	3.45885959	5.86363636	2.96480072	5.04000000	3.23367696
QUEST14	5.84375000	3.21397528	7.27272727	2.54823596	6.28000000	2.79165423
QUEST15	7.75000000	2.01606452	8.13636364	1.80727247	7.64000000	1.95533458
SATIS	0.68750000	0.47092907	0.72727273	0.45584231	0.84000000	0.37416574

154

relationships after counseling. The correlations between the components of counseling under investigation with satisfaction and associated probability values grouped by age are presented in Table 9.5.

Table 9.5 Spearman Correlation Coefficients of CAPS Client Satisfaction Questionnaire Items with Satisfaction and Associated Probability Values by Age

Item	19 and Younger (N = 32)		20–22 (N = 22)		23 and Older (N = 25)	
QUEST1	0.56061	0.0009	0.58161	0.0045	0.71955	0.0001
QUEST2	0.76556	0.0001	0.74138	0.0001	0.65870	0.0003
QUEST3	0.80950	0.0001	0.73439	0.0001	0.56856	0.0030
QUEST4	0.64927	0.0001	0.82769	0.0001	0.52572	0.0070
QUEST5	0.81381	0.0001	0.63417	0.0015	0.52515	0.0070
QUEST6	0.60925	0.0002	0.36000	0.0998	0.33696	0.0995
QUEST7	0.81386	0.0001	0.69922	0.0003	0.77357	0.0001
QUEST8	0.61670	0.0002	0.27846	0.2095	0.61099	0.0012
QUEST9	0.61593	0.0002	0.76726	0.0001	0.55013	0.0044
QUEST10	0.79326	0.0001	0.78525	0.0001	0.39303	0.0519
QUEST11	0.31937	0.0748	0.49665	0.0187	0.70380	0.0001
QUEST12	0.36309	0.0411	0.53954	0.0096	0.73069	0.0001
QUEST13	0.31652	0.0776	-0.28040	0.2062	0.37025	0.0685
QUEST14	0.11041	0.5475	-0.22456	0.3150	0.23140	0.2657
QUEST15	0.77500	0.0001	0.67554	0.0006	0.73459	0.0001
SATIS	0.85281	0.0001	0.80554	0.0001	0.73168	0.0001

In terms of the counselor components, the relationship between feeling "the counselor understood me" (item 3) and satisfaction decreased sharply with age as did the relationship between satisfaction and seeing the counselor as "real" (item 5). Feeling comfortable with the counselor (item 4) appeared most associated with satisfaction for students 20 to 22 years of age and least associated for students 23 and older. This was also the case for seeing the counselor as a "warm person" (item 9). However, the relationship between satisfaction and seeing the counselor as skilled (item 15) was least among students 20 to 22 years old and greatest among students 19 and younger.

As for outcome-related perceptions, the relationship between satisfaction and increased self-understanding (item 1) showed a steady increase with age, whereas "I accomplished what I hoped to" (item 7) showed variability with age. However, the association between satisfaction and the student's assessment that his or her methods of dealing with problems had changed (item 11) increased steadily and impressively with age. The same was true for the outcome perception of being "more certain of my ability to make good decisions" (item 12). These items all allude to a sense of self-trust and confidence that is necessary to function autonomously. It appears that outcome states related to increased autonomy as perceived by the student become more associated with satisfaction as age increases.

Looking at technique-related components, assisting the student in clarifying what is wanted from counseling (item 2) was found to be less associated with satisfaction as age increased, as was helping to clarify how the student has been dealing with frustration (item 6). The relationship between satisfaction and reported counselor encouragement (item 10) decreased with age also, and dramatically so, for students 23 and older. Substantially less association with satisfaction was found for the counselor helping to break the problem down into smaller parts (item 8) for students between 20 and 22. However, relating past family experiences to current situations (item 13) was negatively correlated with satisfaction for students between 20 and 22 but positively correlated with satisfaction for both of the other age groups. Feeling uncomfortable at times (item 14) revealed a similar pattern.

To summarize, the data suggest that for the most part components of counseling stressing the counselor's role in "helping" decrease in relation to satisfaction as age increases and components emphasizing the student's control and actions increase in relation to satisfaction as age increases. Thus, the older the student is, the more the student must feel personal control in the counseling process in order to feel satisfied. With younger students, factors related to the counselor's therapeutic presence (encouragement, skill, authenticity, and being understanding) appear more related to satisfaction. The 20 to 22-year-old students present the interesting picture of being the group most satisfied with counselor warmth and comfort and yet being the group least concerned with counselor skill and family influences in terms of satisfaction with counseling.

COMPARISONS OF THE COMPONENTS OF COUNSELING
BY NUMBER OF SESSIONS ATTENDED

Of this sample 41 students attended between one and
three sessions, 16 attended four to six sessions, ten came
for between seven and nine sessions, four came for between
10 and 12 sessions and ten attended 13 or more sessions.
The mean ratings and standard deviations grouped by the
number of sessions attended appear in Tables 9.6a and 9.6b.
It is evident that the mean satisfaction ratings (item 16)
increased progressively with the number of sessions attended
until the 13 sessions or more category. Seventy percent
of all students coming for between one and three sessions
were at least "quite satisfied" (a rating of seven or higher) while 62 percent of those coming four to six times
were satisfied to the same degree. Eighty percent of the
students coming seven to nine times were at least "quite
satisfied," whereas 100 percent of those coming 10 to 12
times and 80 percent of those attending 13 or more sessions
were at least "quite satisfied." Thus, in looking at both
methods of viewing satisfaction, there was, in general,
increased satisfaction as the number of sessions attended
increased, until the last category.

The more sessions attended, the more the students reported an increase in self-understanding (item 1) as a result
of counseling and an increase in feeling that the counselor
understood them (item 3). The latter did show a .15 decrease
in the mean rating for the 13 or more sessions category.
Obviously, it is probable that feeling understood by the
counselor and thinking that self-understanding was increasing
might influence a student to attend more sessions. The other
items do not increase or decrease consistently regarding the
mean rating with the number of sessions attended. However,
mean ratings for feeling comfortable with the counselor (item
4), perceiving the counselor as authentic (item 5), seeing the
counselor as skilled (item 15), and finding the counselor encouraging (item 10) all increased as the number of sessions
attended increased until the last category of 13 or more sessions. The mean ratings by this group for items 4, 5, 10,
and 15 were lower than the ratings by the 10-12 session group.
Any number of explanations as to why this occurred might be
formulated; however, since seven of the ten students in this
group had attended over 20 sessions, and thus by most defini-
tions their therapy was no longer brief, phenomena more associated with longer-term psychotherapy, such as transference,
might be relevant in explaining this difference.

The correlations between satisfaction and the 15 components of counseling appear in Table 9.7. When grouped by number of sessions attended, no consistent trends were evident

Table 9.6a Mean Ratings and Standard Deviations on CAPS Client Satisfaction Questionnaire Items by Number of Sessions Attended (1-9 sessions)

Item	1-3 Sessions		4-6 Sessions		7-9 Sessions	
	Mean Rating	Standard Deviation	Mean Rating	Standard Deviation	Mean Rating	Standard Deviation
QUEST16	7.29268293	2.24993225	7.68750000	1.95682566	8.20000000	2.09761770
QUEST1	5.17073171	2.10834579	6.25000000	2.51661148	6.30000000	3.46570499
QUEST2	5.95121951	2.35532609	6.56250000	1.93110504	6.50000000	2.46080384
QUEST3	6.24390244	2.29978790	6.87500000	2.15638587	7.00000000	2.62466929
QUEST4	6.65853659	2.25399375	7.18750000	2.31570724	7.20000000	2.39443800
QUEST5	7.78048780	2.07981003	8.18750000	1.72119145	8.60000000	1.83787317
QUEST6	5.51219512	2.81177836	6.25000000	2.90975371	6.40000000	3.09838668
QUEST7	6.39024390	2.63512854	5.62500000	2.33452351	6.90000000	3.28125992
QUEST8	5.65853659	2.42497171	6.37500000	2.55277627	7.50000000	2.32139805
QUEST9	7.60975610	2.20088674	7.62500000	2.24722051	8.30000000	2.00277585
QUEST10	7.39024390	1.96058727	7.56250000	1.99895806	8.30000000	1.33749351
QUEST11	5.70731707	2.73170187	5.62500000	2.24722051	6.30000000	2.75075747
QUEST12	4.82926829	2.94874922	5.31250000	2.08865986	6.40000000	2.50333111
QUEST13	4.29268293	3.02691181	5.50000000	2.68328157	6.70000000	3.36815149
QUEST14	5.65853659	3.04638931	6.62500000	3.13847097	8.20000000	1.39841180
QUEST15	7.41463415	2.26909244	8.00000000	2.00000000	8.00000000	1.05409255
SATIS	0.70731707	0.46064642	0.62500000	0.50000000	0.80000000	0.42163702

Table 9.6b Mean Ratings and Standard Deviations on CAPS
Client Satisfaction Questionnaire Items by Number of
Sessions Attended (10 or more sessions)

	10-12 Sessions (*N* = 4)		*13 or More Sessions* (*N* = 10)	
Item	Mean Rating	Standard Deviation	Mean Rating	Standard Deviation
QUEST16	8.25000000	0.95742711	7.70000000	2.90784380
QUEST1	7.25000000	1.25830574	7.40000000	2.22111083
QUEST2	6.50000000	1.00000000	6.20000000	2.29975844
QUEST3	7.75000000	1.70782513	7.60000000	2.17050941
QUEST4	9.25000000	0.95742711	7.80000000	2.85968141
QUEST5	9.25000000	0.95742711	8.10000000	2.37814120
QUEST6	5.00000000	4.24264069	6.20000000	2.20100987
QUEST7	5.50000000	2.08166600	7.00000000	2.74873708
QUEST8	7.00000000	1.63299316	6.70000000	1.63639169
QUEST9	7.25000000	4.85626743	8.50000000	2.91547595
QUEST10	8.50000000	0.57735027	8.30000000	2.71006355
QUEST11	6.75000000	1.50000000	6.60000000	3.62705880
QUEST12	5.00000000	0.81649658	6.00000000	2.70801280
QUEST13	4.00000000	4.54606057	6.80000000	3.42539535
QUEST14	7.25000000	3.40342964	7.20000000	2.29975844
QUEST15	8.75000000	1.25830574	7.90000000	1.72884033
SATIS	1.00000000	0.00000000	0.80000000	0.42163702

with regard to correlational scores beyond the fact that all
components other than feeling uncomfortable at times (item
14) were always positively correlated to varying degrees with
satisfaction with four exceptions. Perceiving the counselor
as skilled (item 15) showed a negative correlation with
satisfaction for those students attending 10 to 12 sessions
(*N* = 4). The counselor encouraging the student to relate current concerns to past family experiences (item 13) showed a
negative relationship with satisfaction for students attending 13 or more sessions. Encouragement by the counselor that
the situation might improve (item 10) was negatively related
to satisfaction for students attending 10 to 12 sessions.
For the same group of students there was a more noteworthy

Table 9.7 Spearman Correlation Coefficients of CAPS Client
Satisfaction Questionnaire Items with Satisfaction and
Associated Probability Values by Number of Sessions
Attended

Item	*Number of Sessions*				
	1-3	4-6	7-9	10-12	13 or more
QUEST1	0.47933	0.84271	0.67861	0.48420	0.94963
	0.0015	0.0001	0.0310	0.5158	0.0001
QUEST2	0.75757	0.64945	0.75339	0.87039	0.74104
	0.0001	0.0065	0.0119	0.1296	0.0142
QUEST3	0.77339	0.68528	0.68618	0.05096	0.87671
	0.0001	0.0034	0.0285	0.9490	0.0009
QUEST4	0.60683	0.66112	0.69906	0.63636	0.94068
	0.0001	0.0053	0.0245	0.3636	0.0001
QUEST5	0.65518	0.86969	0.80124	0.63636	0.55112
	0.0001	0.0001	0.0053	0.3636	0.0987
QUEST6	0.43411	0.83423	0.20857	0.57443	0.75692
	0.0046	0.0001	0.5631	0.4256	0.0113
QUEST7	0.76034	0.74609	0.89111	0.75262	0.84798
	0.0001	0.0009	0.0005	0.2474	0.0019
QUEST8	0.49990	0.74570	0.36509	0.00000	0.70285
	0.0009	0.0009	0.2996	1.0000	0.0234
QUEST9	0.73045	0.63863	0.59244	0.84238	0.72739
	0.0001	0.0078	0.0711	0.1576	0.0171
QUEST10	0.59121	0.86601	0.72871	-0.30151	0.88687
	0.0001	0.0001	0.0168	0.6985	0.0006
QUEST11	0.29902	0.56283	0.43135	0.98644	0.84069
	0.0575	0.0232	0.2133	0.0136	0.0023
QUEST12	0.35063	0.61269	0.70251	-0.85280	0.93128
	0.0246	0.0116	0.0235	0.1472	0.0001
QUEST13	0.23306	0.08253	0.43406	0.53609	-0.18518
	0.1425	0.7612	0.2101	0.4639	0.6085
QUEST14	-0.17107	0.64181	-0.20455	-0.43476	-0.30572
	0.2849	0.0074	0.5708	0.5652	0.3903
QUEST15	0.82769	0.80062	0.55277	-0.20751	0.61223
	0.0001	0.0002	0.0975	0.7925	0.0599
SATIS	0.83248	0.89431	0.80403	0.00000	0.85187
	0.0001	0.0001	0.0051	1.0000	0.0018

negative relationship between satisfaction and reporting that confidence in decision-making ability had improved through counseling.

One possible approach to this piece of data would be to examine which components of counseling were most positively associated with satisfaction at each phase of the counseling process. Given a relatively homogeneous population, it would appear valuable to look at this despite the fact that it is not a true repeated measures design. However, the repeated measures design would have other inherent methodological problems concerning the effects of the repeated measures themselves. During the first three counseling sessions the most valued (most highly correlated with satisfaction) non-outcome-related components were the counselor being seen as skilled, understanding, helping with goal clarification, and warmth.

For those attending four to six sessions, the nonoutcome components most related to satisfaction were the student's perception of the counselor as authentic, encouraging, helping to clarify how frustration had been dealt with, and being skilled. Students coming for seven to nine times found counselor authenticity, assisted goal clarification, encouragement, and the perception of being comfortable with the counselor as most related to satisfaction. For those attending 10 to 12 sessions, counselor-assisted goal clarification and warmth were important, but the only item that correlated with satisfaction to the statistically significant degree of $p < .05$ was the outcome-related item of changing methods of dealing with problems. Consequently it appears that this group of four students was quite idiosyncratic.

Those students attending 13 or more sessions found feeling comfortable with the counselor, counselor encouragement, and feeling understood by the counselor to be most associated with satisfaction. Although certain elements were more associated with satisfaction than others by students attending different numbers of sessions, the relationship variables of warmth, understanding, authenticity, and comfort were almost always significant in relation to satisfaction. Perceived counselor skill faded in importance as the number of sessions attended increased, until the last category, where it again was highly related to satisfaction. The cognitive intervention components of goal clarification and encouragement appear by and large to have been consistently valued and the clarification of methods used to deal with frustration was significantly related to satisfaction except for those attending between seven and 12 sessions.

The outcome variable most consistently and highly related to satisfaction was "Accomplishing what I had hoped to." The others (items 1, 11, and 12) showed a generally positive but variable relation to satisfaction when viewed by the number

of sessions attended. Again the relating of past family
experiences to current concerns for the most part showed a
weak relationship with satisfaction, and a fairly consistent
negative relationship between feeling uncomfortable at times
and satisfaction was found across the number-of-sessions-
attended categories.

It is interesting to note that a different component of
counseling was most highly correlated with satisfaction for
each of the number-of-sessions-attended groups. However,
since there were different students in each group, it would
be erroneous to conclude from the data that specific components of counseling are best utilized at a particular phase
of counseling. Nevertheless, it might be hypothesized that
students who find a particular component of counseling most
satisfying are more likely to attend a certain number of
sessions. Thus, students who expect to attend fewer sessions
may value counselor expertise most highly as it fits their
personal model of what counseling is or should be like and
how they wish to see themselves using it. Therefore, if the
counselor can discover how many sessions the student thinks
s/he might attend, then it may be possible to utilize more
fully the components of counseling that will most satisfy a
particular student. However, in viewing the data at hand,
the most important differences do not appear to be associated
with the number of sessions attended. Subgroup analyses by
age and sex should reveal the primary relevant differences.

SUBGROUP ANALYSES

For further comparisons, the sample will be divided by
age and sex such that there are three groups of women: 19
and younger ($N = 24$), 20 to 22 year olds ($N = 17$), and those
23 and older ($N = 11$); and three corresponding groups of men:
($N = 8$), ($N = 5$), and ($N = 14$). The small number of men 20 to
22 makes the findings related to this group quite questionable. The responses to questions 17, 18, and 19 indicate
that there was an increase in the percentage of women rating
academic performance as "better" after counseling as age
increased. Men, on the other hand, showed a decrease with
age in the percentage reporting "better" academic performance
after counseling. The percentage of women reporting "better"
social relationships after counseling also increased as age
increased. Again the percentage of men reporting the situation to be "better" after counseling decreased with age.
Despite these trends, the percentage of men rating academic
performance and social relationships as "better" after counseling was greater than the percentage of women reporting to
be "better" in the age categories of 19 and younger and 20 to
22. The correlations of the components of counseling with

satisfaction for these groups appear in Table 9.8a and 9.8b.
It is evident that a relationship between age and sex exists
for feeling understood by counselor (item 3) such that the
correlation between satisfaction and feeling understood
decreases with age for women and increases with age for men.
Age and sex appear to be related to the belief that self-understanding (item 1) was improved as a result of counseling in a
curvilinear manner such that for women the strongest correlation occurred in the 20 to 22 age category while for men the
weakest correlation occurred in that age category. The same
is true for the correlation of counselor warmth (item 9) with
satisfaction. The correlation between feeling uncomfortable
at times (item 14) with satisfaction was most negative for
women 20 to 22 years old, yet for men the correlation was
highest and significantly so, during these years.

Relating past family experiences to current concerns
appears to have been affected by both sex and age in that the
correlation with satisfaction was slightly positive for women
19 and under but very high and significantly positive for men
in this age group. For women between 20 and 22, there was a
negative relationship between the two items while for men in
this age category the correlation was highly positive and
statistically significant. For women 23 and older there was
a strong positive correlation between the two, although the
relationship was not quite significant at the $p < .05$ level.
However, the men in this older age group showed only a
slightly positive correlation that was not significant between the two items. Thus, in general, relating past family
experiences to current concerns was most valued by men (particularly those younger than 23).

Likewise the correlation of satisfaction with a self-
perceived change in the methods of dealing with problems
(item 11) was also highly influenced by sex. In each age
category the correlation with satisfaction was higher for men
than women. The association between satisfaction and encouragement lessens progressively with age for both men and women
suggesting that the importance of encouragement in counseling
is primarily age-related. Although encouragement was considerably more related to satisfaction for women than men
when a comparison by sex alone was made, if age is also taken
into account, it is apparent that this difference is slight
for students 19 and younger. Moreover, for students 23 and
older, men valued encouragement more than women. Concerning
the reported increase in certainty of the ability to make
good decisions (item 12) as related to satisfaction, the
relationship between these two items increased with age for
women, whereas for men the relationship was strongest with
the youngest age group and weakest for 20 to 22 year olds.
There is great variability by age within the male and female
groups, such that both sex and age are important as influ-

Table 9.8a   Spearman Correlation Coefficients of CAPS Client Satisfaction Questionnaire Items with Satisfaction and Associated Probability Values by Age and Sex: Females

Item	19 and Younger (N = 24)		20-22 (N = 17)		23 and Older (N = 11)	
QUEST1	0.53594	0.0070	0.56065	0.0192	0.46568	0.1489
QUEST2	0.77004	0.0001	0.71576	0.0012	0.40996	0.2105
QUEST3	0.87593	0.0001	0.70234	0.0017	0.43538	0.1808
QUEST4	0.74117	0.0001	0.82102	0.0001	0.32725	0.3259
QEUST5	0.85843	0.0001	0.60395	0.0102	0.23578	0.4852
QUEST6	0.62296	0.0012	0.39706	0.1145	0.71686	0.0130
QUEST7	0.78806	0.0001	0.70076	0.0017	0.58233	0.0601
QUEST8	0.61820	0.0013	0.26258	0.3086	0.56564	0.0697
QUEST9	0.60121	0.0019	0.75703	0.0004	0.26667	0.4280
QUEST10	0.80342	0.0001	0.76792	0.0003	0.11016	0.7471
QUEST11	0.23252	0.2742	0.52627	0.0300	0.38615	0.2408
QUEST12	0.26551	0.2099	0.65165	0.0046	0.73973	0.0093
QUEST13	0.16410	0.4435	-0.39197	0.1197	0.53572	0.0894
QUEST14	-0.05991	0.7809	-0.23873	0.3561	0.41936	0.1992
QUEST15	0.79276	0.0001	0.65286	0.0045	0.80180	0.0030
SATIS	0.83993	0.0001	0.79266	0.0001	0.00000	1.0000

164

Table 9.8b Spearman Correlation Coefficients of CAPS Client Satisfaction Questionnaire Items with Satisfaction and Associated Probability Values by Age and Sex: Males

Item	19 and Younger ($N = 8$)		20-22 ($N = 5$)		23 and Older ($N = 14$)	
QUEST1	0.70998	0.0485	0.66667	0.2191	0.79094	0.0008
QUEST2	0.79721	0.0178	0.66989	0.2160	0.69122	0.0062
QUEST3	0.55460	0.1537	0.64169	0.2432	0.73685	0.0026
QUEST4	0.36403	0.3753	0.32733	0.5908	0.68534	0.0068
QUEST5	0.66837	0.0700	0.41251	0.4901	0.57628	0.0310
QUEST6	0.68593	0.0604	0.64752	0.2375	0.16357	0.5763
QUEST7	0.90950	0.0017	0.07143	0.9091	0.85652	0.0001
QUEST8	0.78139	0.0220	0.10249	0.8697	0.59436	0.0250
QUEST9	0.86053	0.0061	0.53452	0.3534	0.70631	0.0047
QUEST10	0.84799	0.0078	0.64286	0.2420	0.42189	0.1329
QUEST11	0.67178	0.0681	0.97943	0.0035	0.77470	0.0011
QUEST12	0.75019	0.0320	0.32733	0.5908	0.71867	0.0038
QUEST13	0.85181	0.0073	0.96312	0.0085	0.28594	0.3217
QUEST14	0.81981	0.0127	0.89521	0.0401	0.07492	0.7991
QUEST15	0.79570	0.0182	0.42258	0.4784	0.69989	0.0053
SATIS	0.90562	0.0020	0.00000	1.0000	0.80298	0.0005

165

encing factors for this variable. Thus for males, achieving increased confidence in decision-making ability through counseling is more related to satisfaction than it is for women in the group of students 19 and younger. However, the opposite was true opposite was true for students between 20 and 22 years of age, and for students 23 and older the relationship was quite similar.

The relationship of counselor assistance in breaking the problem down into smaller parts (item 8) to satisfaction appears to be primarily influenced by age. For both sexes the realtionship is significantly positive and strong for students in the youngest age group. The relationship then lessens markedly for students in the next age category. However, students in the oldest age group once again show a strong relationship between the two items.

The correlation between satisfaction and accomplishing what the student hoped to (item 7) is related to age for women since the correlation weakens as age increases among women. However, men 20 to 22 show a surprisingly weak correlation between satisfaction and accomplishing what they hoped to. Nevertheless, for the most part, older students do not associate satisfaction with services received and accomplishing what they had hoped to as much younger students do. This may be a reflection of older students being more satisfied in general with services received. Further, higher satisfaction ratings were more associated with higher ratings on all of the outcome-related components (items 1, 7, 11, and 12) for men than women. This suggests that a perceived increase in self-understanding, accomplishing what the student hoped to, changing methods of dealing with problems, and becoming more certain of the ability to make good decisions as a result of counseling is more important vis à vis satisfaction for men than women. Thus the possibility again emerges that men and women may want somewhat different things from counseling.

The relationship between satisfaction and counselor-assisted clarification of means used in dealing with frustration (item 6) appears to be related to both sex and age in that the correlations with satisfaction are stronger for men who are 22 and younger, women 23 and older, and women 19 and younger.

Satisfaction and perceived counselor authenticity (item 5) were also related in such a way that both age and sex affected the relationship. Women showed a progressive decrease in the strength of the relationship as age increased. Thus older women found it less important to see the counselor as authentic than did younger women. However, for men the relationship varied with age so that seeing the counselor as authentic was highly associated with satisfaction for both the youngest and the oldest age groups but less so for men in

the 20 to 22 age group. Further, the relationship between
the two items for students under 23 was greater for women
whereas for students 23 and older the relationship between
satisfaction and perceived counselor authenticity was greater
for men.

The correlation between feeling comfortable with the
counselor (item 4) and satisfaction again reveals that both
age and sex appear to be related variables since feeling
comfortable with the counselor was more related to satisfaction for men than for women among students 23 and older.
However, for students younger than 23, comfort with the counselor was more related to satisfaction for women. Thus the
relationship between these two items increased with age for
women until the age category of 23 and older, at which point
the relationship was weakest. On the other hand, for men the
relationship decreased in strength with age until the category of 23 and older and the relationship was strongest for
these men. Feeling comfortable with the counselor was significantly correlated with satisfaction for males 23 and older
while for females the correlation was significant for those
22 and younger. This is consistent with the findings regarding feeling uncomfortable at times (item 14).

Counselor-assisted clarification of the goals of counseling (item 2) was related to satisfaction in a way that also
revealed effects by both age and sex. For women the relationship between counselor-assisted clarification of goals (item
2) and satisfaction weakened as age increased, while for men
the same trend appeared across the first two age categories,
but a slight increase in the correlation was found for men in
the 23 and older age group. Nevertheless, the relationship
was statistically significant for women 22 and younger but
was also significant for men in the youngest and oldest age
categories although the relationship was not significant for
those in the 20- to 22-year-old category.

IMPLICATIONS FOR TREATMENT

If it is assumed that the data has relevance for treatment with similar university populations, some interesting
points can be gleaned. For women 19 and under the most
important components of counseling, based on the correlations
with satisfaction, appear to be feeling understood by the
counselor and seeing the counselor as authentic, encouraging,
and skilled. Women between 20 and 22 found feeling comfortable with the counselor, as well as the counselor's being
encouraging, warm, and helping to clarify the goals of counseling as most related to satisfaction. It was found that
women in the age group of 23 and older found perceived counselor skill, becoming more certain of the ability to make

good decisions, counselor-assisted clarification of "how I had been dealing with frustration" and "accomplishing what I had hoped to" as most related to satisfaction.

Men 19 and younger associated "accomplishing what I had hoped to," counselor warmth, the relating of past family experiences to current situations, and encouragement most related to satisfaction. The components found to correlate most highly with satisfaction for 20 to 22-year-old men were perceiving a change in methods of dealing with problems, relating current situations to past family experiences, feeling uncomfortable at times, and counselor-assisted clarification of what was wanted from counseling. The ratings of men 23 and older found to correlate most with satisfaction were accomplishing what was hoped for, increasing self-understanding, changing methods of dealing with problems, and feeling understood by the counselor.

To summarize, the variables of sex and age appear to influence the relationship between certain components of counseling and satisfaction. For some components the relationship was primarily influenced by sex. This was the case for perceiving an increase in self-understanding as a result of counseling. Perceived counselor skill appears to have been primarily affected by sex also, if probability levels are taken into account, because the relationship to satisfaction is stronger for women in each age category. The correlations of the remaining components with satisfaction appear to have been influenced by a relationship between sex and age. For the most part, satisfaction was less associated with components of counseling emphasizing the counselor's helping activity as age increased, such as was found with item 10.

Women 23 and older and men between 20 and 22 had the fewest significant correlations between the different components of counseling and satisfaction while women in the oldest age group appeared quite different from those in the other two age groups regarding what was associated with satisfaction for them. On the other hand, the correlations between the components of counseling for men 23 and older with satisfaction were more similar to men 19 and younger than to men between 20 and 22. Since there were only five students in this latter category, hypotheses based on the data for this group must be seen largely as conjecture. It might be hypothesized, based on the data, that women 23 and older (in all likelihood graduate/professional students) and men between 20 and 22 need to attribute the cause of improvement more to themselves than to the counselor or the counseling process. It is possible that older male undergraduates and graduate/professional female students have greater interest in seeing themselves as autonomous and independent than the other groups of students.

In conclusion, the variables of sex and age often influence the components of counseling most highly correlated with satisfaction. For some components sex appears to be the dominant factor influencing the correlation with satisfaction, while for other components age appears to be dominant. A third group of components is most influenced by a relationship between both sex and age. Although a university population may be relatively homogeneous in many ways, effective work with students in individual psychosocial counseling can be enhanced when treatment is viewed in the context of specific student variables such as sex and age.

REFERENCES

Bent, R., D. Putnam, D. Kiesler, and S. Nowicki. "Correlates of Successful and Unsuccessful Psychotherapy." *Journal of Consulting and Clinical Psychology* 44 (1976):149.

Bergin, A. and S. Garfield, editors. *Handbook of Psychotherapy and Behavior Change: An Empirical Analysis*. 2nd ed. New York: Wiley, 1978.

Gelso, C. and D. Johnson. *Explorations in Time Limited Counseling and Psychotherapy*. New York: Teachers College Press, 1983.

Heppner, P. and M. Heesacker. "Perceived Counselor Characteristics, Client Expectations, and Client Satisfaction with Counseling." *Journal of Counseling Psychology* 30 (1983): 31-39.

Horenstein, D., B. Houston, and S. Holmes. "Clients', Therapists' and Judges' Evaluations of Psychotherapy." *Journal of Counseling Psychology* 20 (1973):149-153.

Jansen, D. and M. Aldrich. "State Hospital Psychiatric Patients Evaluate Their Treatment Teams." *Hospital and Community Psychiatry* 24 (1973):768-770.

Kline, F., A. Adrian, and M. Spevak. "Patients Evaluate Therapists." *Archives of General Psychiatry* 31 (1974): 113-116.

Linden, J., S. Stone, and B. Shertzer. "Development and Evaluation of an Inventory for Rating Counseling." *Personnel and Guidance Journal* 43 (1965):276-277.

Newton, F. and R. Caple. "Client and Counselor Preferences for Counselor Behavior in the Interview." *Journal of College Student Personnel* 15 (1974):220-224.

Resnick, H. "Consumer Satisfaction: Its Utility for Coun-
   seling Services." Paper presented at the 86th Annual
   Meeting of the American Psychological Association, 1978,
   Toronto.

Rogers, C. *Client-Centered Therapy: Its Current Practice,
   Implications, and Theory.* Boston: Houghton Mifflin,
   1951.

Strong, S. "Counseling: An Interpersonal Influence Process."
   Journal of Counseling Psychology 15 (1968):215-224.

Strupp, H. *Psychotherapy: Clinical, Research, and Theoretical Issues.* New York: Jason Aronson, 1973.

Strupp, H., R. Rox, and K. Lessler. *Patients View Their Psychotherapy.* Baltimore: Johns Hopkins Press, 1969.

Weber, D. and D. Tilley. "Patients' Evaluations of the
   Mental Health Service at a Health Sciences Campus."
   Journal of the American College Health Association 29
   (1981):193-194.

Zung, W.W.K. "A Self-Rating Depression Scale." *Archives of
   General Psychiatry* 12 (1965):63-70.

---. "A Rating Instrument for Anxiety Disorders." *Psychosomatics* 12 (1971):371-379.

---, C.D. Richards, and M.J. Short. "Self-Rating Depression
   Scale in an Outpatient Clinic." *Archives of General
   Psychiatry* 13 (1965):508.

APPENDIX A

Zung Self-Rating Depression Scale (Items 1-20)

Zung Self-Rating Anxiety Scale (Items 20-40)

	None or a little of the time	Some of the time	Good part of the time	Most or all of the time
1. I feel down-hearted and blue				
2. Morning is when I feel the best				
3. I have crying spells or feel like it				
4. I have trouble sleeping at night				
5. I eat as much as I used to				
6. I still enjoy sex				
7. I notice that I am losing weight				
8. I have trouble with constipation				
9. My heart beats faster than usual				
10. I get tired for no reason				
11. My mind is as clear as it used to be				
12. I find it easy to do the things I used to				
13. I am restless and can't keep still				
14. I feel hopeful about the future				
15. I am more irritable than usual				
16. I find it easy to make decisions				
17. I feel that I am useful and needed				
18. My life is pretty full				
19. I feel that others would be better off if I were dead				
20. I still enjoy the things I used to do				

21. I feel more nervous and anxious than usual
22. I feel afraid for no reason at all
23. I get upset easily or feel panicky
24. I feel like I'm falling apart and going to pieces
25. I feel that everything is all right and nothing bad will happen
26. My arms and legs shake and tremble
27. I am bothered by headaches, neck and back pains
28. I feel weak and get tired easily
29. I feel calm and can sit still easily
30. I can feel my heart beating fast
31. I am bothered by dizzy spells
32. I have fainting spells or feel like it
33. I can breathe in and out easily
34. I get feelings of numbness and tingling in my fingers, toes
35. I am bothered by stomach aches or indigestion
36. I have to empty my bladder often
37. My hands are usually dry and warm
38. My face gets hot and blushes
39. I fall asleep easily and get a good night's rest
40. I have nightmares

APPENDIX B

CAPS Client Satisfaction Questionnaire

Please respond to the following questions by rating on a scale from one to ten how true the statement is of your personal counseling experience at CAPS.

(1.) I understand myself better as a result of counseling.

1	2	3	4	5	6	7	8	9	10
Not at all true			Somewhat true			Quite true			Extremely true

(2.) The counselor helped me clarify what I wanted to get out of counseling.

1	2	3	4	5	6	7	8	9	10
Not at all true			Somewhat true			Quite true			Extremely true

(3.) I felt the counselor understood me.

1	2	3	4	5	6	7	8	9	10
Not at all true			Somewhat true			Quite true			Extremely true

(4.) I felt comfortable with the counselor.

1	2	3	4	5	6	7	8	9	10
Not at all true			Somewhat true			Quite true			Extremely true

(5.) The counselor seemed to be authentic or "real".

1	2	3	4	5	6	7	8	9	10
Not at all true			Somewhat true			Quite true			Extremely true

(6.) The counselor helped me clarify how I had been dealing with frustration.

1	2	3	4	5	6	7	8	9	10
Not at all true			Somewhat true			Quite true			Extremely true

(7.) I accomplished what I had hoped to by coming to CAPS.

1	2	3	4	5	6	7	8	9	10
Not at all true			Somewhat true			Quite true			Extremely true

(8.)   The counselor helped me to break the problem down into smaller parts.

1	2	3	4	5	6	7	8	9	10
Not at all true			Somewhat true			Quite true			Extremely true

(9.)   The counselor seemed to be a warm person.

1	2	3	4	5	6	7	8	9	10
Not at all true			Somewhat true			Quite true			Extremely true

(10.)   The counselor encouraged me to believe that I could improve my situation.

1	2	3	4	5	6	7	8	9	10
Not at all true			Somewhat true			Quite true			Extremely true

(11.)   My methods of dealing with the problems I face have changed as a result of counseling.

1	2	3	4	5	6	7	8	9	10
Not at all true			Somewhat true			Quite true			Extremely true

(12.)   Through counseling I have become more certain of my ability to make good decisions.

1	2	3	4	5	6	7	8	9	10
Not at all true			Somewhat true			Quite true			Extremely true

(13.)   The counselor encouraged me to relate my current concerns to past experiences with my family.

1	2	3	4	5	6	7	8	9	10
Not at all true			Somewhat true			Quite true			Extremely true

(14)   At times talking about my situation was uncomfortable.

1	2	3	4	5	6	7	8	9	10
Not at all true			Somewhat true			Quite true			Extremely true

(15.)   The counselor impressed me as a skilled counselor.

1	2	3	4	5	6	7	8	9	10
Not at all true			Somewhat true			Quite true			Extremely true

(16.) In summary, I am satisfied with the services I received at CAPS.

1	2	3	4	5	6	7	8	9	10
Not at all true			Somewhat true			Quite true			Extremely true

Please check either 1, 2, or 3 for the next three questions.

(17.) Have you sought counseling elsewhere since your experience at CAPS?

____ 1) Yes, at the recommendation of the counselor

____ 2) Yes, not due to recommendation of the counselor

____ 3) No

(18.) How does your current academic performance compare to your performance prior to coming to CAPS?

____ 1) The Same

____ 2) Better

____ 3) Worse

(19.) How does the quality of your current relationships with others compare to the quality of them prior to coming to CAPS?

____ 1) The same

____ 2) Better

____ 3) Worse

Author Index

Subject Index

About the Authors and Editors

JOHN C. BARROW is Staff Psychologist and Coordinator of Career Counseling, Structured Groups and Outreach Programming at Counseling and Psychological Services, Duke University. He is also Clinical Assistant Professor, Department of Psychiatry, Duke University Medical Center.

Dr. Barrow is the author of *Cognitive Approaches in Student Development Counseling and Programming* and is a Diplomate of The American Board of Professional Psychology.

CONRAD C. FULKERSON is Psychiatric Consultant to The Division of General Medicine, Department of Medicine, Duke University Medical Center where he is also Clinical Assistant Professor in the Department of Psychiatry. Dr. Fulkerson is a specialist in both psychiatry and internal medicine and was formerly Staff Psychiatrist, Counseling and Psychological Services, Duke University.

CAROL A. MOORE is Staff Psychologist and Coordinator of Career Counseling at The Counseling and Testing Service at North Texas State University where she is also Assistant Professor, Department of Psychology. Dr. Moore completed her internship at Counseling and Psychological Services, Duke University and has served as Staff Psychologist at the Counseling Center of Virginia Polytechnic Institute and State University in Blacksburg.

JANE CLARK MOORMAN, a clinical social worker, is an Associate in the Department of Psychiatry, Duke University Medical Center. She has been Director of Counseling and Psychological Services, Duke University, since its formation in 1977, and prior to that was Director of the Student Mental Health Service, Duke University.

Ms. Moorman is also Clinical Assistant Professor, Smith College School for Social Work, and a member of the Academy of Certified Social Workers.

ROLFFS S. PINKERTON is Staff Psychologist, Coordinator of Training and Consultation, and Director of the Psychology Internship Program at Counseling and Psychological Services, Duke University. Dr. Pinkerton is an adjunct Lecturer in the Department of Psychology, Duke University and a Diplomate of The American Board of Professional Psychology.

W. J. KENNETH ROCKWELL is an Assistant Professor in the Department of Psychiatry and Medical Director of the Eating Disorders Program, Duke University Medical Center. He is Psychiatrist at Counseling and Psychological Services, Duke

University, and is a former Director of the Student Mental Health Service at both Duke University and the University of Alabama, Tuscaloosa.

Dr. Rockwell is a former N.I.M.H. Fellow in Student Mental Health at Georgetown University and is a Fellow in both The American Psychiatric Association and The American College Health Association. He is a graduate of Washington and Lee University and Duke University Medical School.

ELINOR T. ROY, a clinical social worker, is the Assistant Director of Counseling and Psychological Services. She is Clinical Associate in the Department of Psychiatry, Duke University Medical Center.

Ms. Roy is a former President of the North Carolina Society for Clinical Social Work and a member of the Academy of Certified Social Workers.

JOSEPH E. TALLEY is Staff Psychologist and Coordinator of Research, Program Evaluation and Testing at Counseling and Psychological Services, Duke University. He is also Clinical Associate in the Department of Psychiatry, Duke University Medical Center.

Dr. Talley is co-author with Dr. Lawrence H. Henning of *Study Skills: Establishing a Comprehensive Program at the College Level* and is co-editor with Dr. Rockwell of *Counseling and Psychotherapy Services for University Students*. He received a B.A. from the University of Richmond (Virginia), an M.A. from Radford College (Virginia), a Ph.D. from the University of Virginia, and did graduate study at Temple University and Duke University.